P9-EEU-635

SOCIAL PROBLEMS AND SOCIAL POLICY:
The American Experience

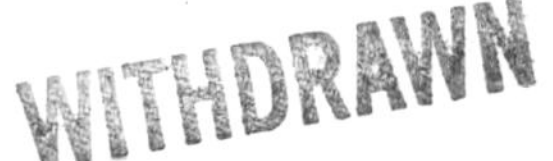

This is a volume in the Arno Press Series

SOCIAL PROBLEMS AND SOCIAL POLICY: The American Experience

See last pages of this volume for a complete list of titles.

MENTAL DISEASE AND SOCIAL WELFARE

By

HORATIO M. POLLOCK

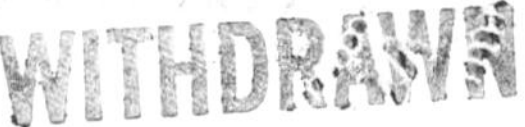

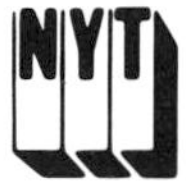

ARNO PRESS
A New York Times Company
New York — 1976

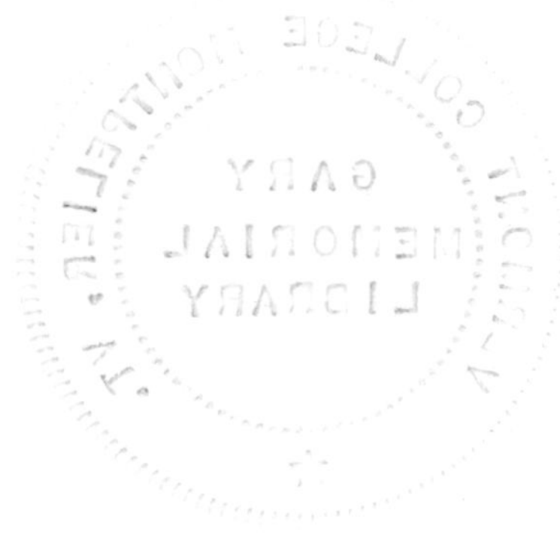

Editorial Supervision: SHEILA MEHLMAN

Reprint Edition 1976 by Arno Press Inc.

Reprinted from a copy in the Princeton University Library

SOCIAL PROBLEMS AND SOCIAL POLICY: The American Experience
ISBN for complete set: 0-405-07474-3
See last pages of this volume for titles.

Manufactured in the United States of America

Library of Congress Cataloging in Publication Data

Pollock, Horatio Milo, 1868-1950.
Mental disease and social welfare.

(Social problems and social policy--the American experience)
Reprint of the ed. published by State Hospitals Press, Utica, N.Y.
Includes bibliographies.
1. Social psychiatry--United States. 2. Mental illness--United States--Statistics. 3. Mental illness--New York (State)--Statistics. 4. Mental illness--Peru. I. Title. II. Series.
RC455.P62 1976 362.2'0973 75-17237
ISBN 0-405-07506-5

MENTAL DISEASE AND SOCIAL WELFARE

By

HORATIO M. POLLOCK

DIRECTOR OF MENTAL HYGIENE STATISTICS
NEW YORK STATE DEPARTMENT OF MENTAL HYGIENE
FORMER EDITOR OF THE PSYCHIATRIC QUARTERLY

STATE HOSPITALS PRESS
UTICA, NEW YORK
1941

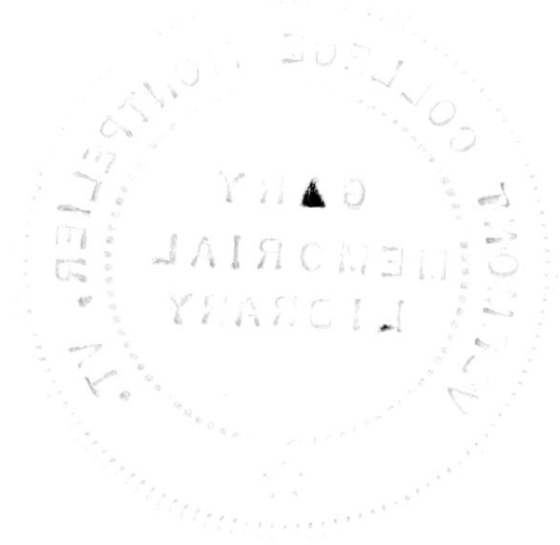

FOREWORD

Coming to the New York State Hospital Commission as statistician and editor in 1911, after teaching sociology and economics in Union College, the author was deeply impressed by the unfavorable influence exerted on society by mental disorders. He early recognized that institutional care of the mentally ill was a rapidly growing problem and that sooner or later it would have to be dealt with in a large way. He witnessed with gratification the establishment of clinics, the employment of social workers, the paroling of patients and the expansion of the mental hygiene movement. He shared the prevailing optimism that the increase in mental hospital population might be checked and that mental illness would eventually be lessened. He became actively interested in the work of the National Committee for Mental Hygiene and served as consultant in the committee's work of establishing a uniform system of statistics of mental disorders throughout the United States. His service in the Division of Psychiatry in the office of the Surgeon-General of the Army in 1917, and his work as adviser to the Federal Census Bureau in the institution census of 1923, confirmed his previous conviction that mental disease constituted an enormous social problem that would be solved only with great difficulty.

From time to time as opportunity was afforded, the author made special research studies. Some of these were prepared for administrative purposes while others were designed to contribute to psychiatric knowledge and to furnish a basis for preventive work. Several of the studies were presented at meetings of national and international associations. In response to numerous requests a group of the studies dealing with important phases of mental disease were selected for this volume. Each chapter comprises a complete study.

The work in the main deals with phases of mental disease that have a direct bearing on social welfare and the problem of the treatment and prevention of mental disorders. Although based on statistics, the larger part of the studies are not primarily statistical; rather, they apply facts gathered from statistics to the several problems discussed.

The studies are now republished in book form to make them available to a wider circle of readers and to make accessible to students and research workers the reference material they contain.

No attempt has been made to supply current statistical data in place of those originally compiled in the several studies. The value of the work will be found in the principles and relations discussed and not in the figures cited. Statistics may show permanent relations although numbers change from day to day.

The author gratefully acknowledges his indebtedness to his coworkers and others, as follows:

To Dr. Benjamin Malzberg, for collaboration in the preparation of the chapter on "Expectation of Mental Disease";

To Mary A. Cooney, Gertrude M. Mack and Ruth Young Hurst, for stenographic and statistical assistance;

To Dr. Clarence B. Farrar, for permission to republish articles that had originally appeared in the American Journal of Psychiatry;

To Dr. George S. Stevenson, for permission to republish articles that originally appeared in Mental Hygiene;

To Dr. Richard H. Hutchings, for permission to republish articles that had originally appeared in the Psychiatric Quarterly;

To Dr. Honorio Delgado, for historical data relating to mental disease in Peru;

To Commissioners William J. Tiffany and Frederick W. Parsons, for their advice and encouragement and for facilitating the preparation of the several studies.

Horatio M. Pollock.

CONTENTS

To
DOCTOR WILLIAM J. TIFFANY
New York State Commissioner of Mental Hygiene,
in recognition of his distinguished service for
the mentally ill, his skillful administration
of mental hospitals, and his continuous
interest in psychiatric and statis-
tical research.

CHAPTER I

Introduction: Social Significance of Mental Disease*

Mental disease has a prominent place among the factors that unfavorably affect the population of all civilized countries. It is fitting therefore that a communication concerning the relation of mental disease to the welfare of society be presented to this Congress.†

The data set forth herein relate in part to the United States and other countries but principally to New York State, as such State is a cosmopolitan commonwealth and has comprehensive comparative statistics of mental disease covering a long series of years.

The following topics are discussed:

1. The prevalence of mental disease;
2. The incidence of mental disease;
3. The expectation of mental disease;
4. Death rates and life expectancy of mental patients;
5. Economic loss due to mental disease;
6. The relation of mental disease to marriage and reproduction;
7. The relation of mental disease to suicide and crime;
8. The future of mental disease.

1. Prevalence of Mental Disease

The prevalence of mental disease varies widely in the several countries of the civilized world and also in different sections of the same country. In certain countries satisfactory data are available relative to mental patients in hospitals, but practically no information is obtainable concerning mentally diseased persons living in the community. The United States Census Bureau from 1850 to 1890 made at 10-year intervals five attempts to enumerate the insane both within and without institutions. The undertaking was not wholly successful. Insanity bore a stigma and was a mysterious affliction. Families could not be expected to brand unfavorably any of their members and enumerators could hardly be considered competent to distinguish between the sane and the insane.

*Presented to †World Population Congress held in Paris, July 28-31, 1937.

The matter was further complicated by the lack of a clear understanding of the dividing lines between mental disease, mental defect and epilepsy. In 1880, the reports of enumerators were supplemented by data collected from physicians throughout the country. When all duplicates were eliminated, it was found that about four-ninths of the total insane were in special institutions for mental cases and five-ninths were outside of such institutions. In 1890 the Census Bureau made its last attempt to enumerate mental patients in the community, but has continued to collect from time to time statistics concerning mental patients in institutions. Since 1926, censuses of such patients have been taken annually. The data thus compiled show a rapidly rising trend in mental patients in institutions and in the rate of mental patients per 100,000 of population. Such rate on January 1, 1936 was 325.7, as compared with 204.2 in 1910, 245.0 in 1923 and 310.5 in 1934. In 1930, according to data collected by Frederick W. Brown, covering 32 countries, rates of mental patients in institutions per 100,000 population varied from 97.5 in Czechoslovakia to 479.3 in the Union of South Africa.

In the United States it has been observed that the states that make adequate provision for mental patients have the highest rates. New York State and Massachusetts both have more than 500 mental patients per 100,000 of population.

Mental disease is more prevalent in cities than in rural districts, and most prevalent in the largest cities. In Manhattan Borough of Greater New York the rate of mental patients under treatment in hospitals in 1936 exceeded 1,000 per 100,000.

Mental disease creates by far the greatest institutional problem with which the State or nation must deal. In New York State on June 30, 1936, there were 68,218 resident patients under treatment in mental hospitals, as compared with 31,908 patients in general hospitals, 7,627 in tuberculosis hospitals and 5,857 in all other types of hospitals, a total of 45,392. On the same date the aggregate prison and jail population of the State was 20,726. It will be observed that mental patients exceeded all other hospital patients combined by over 50 per cent, and were more than three times as numerous as the prison and jail population.

2. Incidence of Mental Disease

There are no complete records pertaining to the annual incidence of mental disease. The best available index is the annual rate of first admissions to hospitals for mental disease. As would be expected, such rate varies considerably from time to time and from place to place. In the several states of the United States a variation from less than 40 to over 100 per 100,000 of population is found. Similar variations are observed in the several countries for which data are available. No definite data exist relative to the many mild cases of mental disorder which occur in the community each year but which do not require treatment in a mental hospital. It is probable that these mild cases outnumber the severe ones that go to mental hospitals.

The rate of incidence as calculated from the first admissions to mental hospitals appears to be gradually increasing, but not so rapidly as the rate of patients under treatment. Most marked increases are found in the arteriosclerotic, alcoholic and dementia præcox groups.

3. Expectation of Mental Disease

A more comprehensive view of the relation of mental disease to the population is shown by data concerning the expectation of mental disease. By the term "expectation of mental disease" is meant the proportion of the population that may be expected to undergo treatment in a hospital for mental disease at some period of life. In 1920, the expectation of mental disease for persons born in New York State was 4.5 per cent.* Among males the expectation was 4.7 per cent and among females, 4.3. Expressed as a ratio, the expectation of mental disease was 1 to 22 for both sexes combined. In other words 1 in 22 of the persons born in the State would be expected to develop serious mental disease and undergo treatment therefor in a mental hospital at some period of life. Since 1920, there has been a notable increase in the incidence of mental disease in New York State. It may therefore be safely estimated that the expectation of mental disease has risen therein to at least 1 to 20. Apparently this is merely the continuation of a trend that has been rising during several generations.

A recent study of the expectation of mental disease in New York

*See Chapter II.

City in 1930 shows the rate of expectation at birth to be 5.7 per cent for males and 5.5 per cent for females; or in ratios, 1 to 17.5 for males, and 1 to 18 for females. When we consider that these data relating to expectation include only hospital cases of mental disease and that mild cases of mental disease that do not reach mental hospitals are probably as numerous as hospital cases, it becomes reasonably certain that at least one-tenth of the population is now or will be afflicted by mental disease.

4. Death Rates and Life Expectancy of Mental Patients

Serious mental disease is a major calamity to the afflicted individual. Only 15 to 20 per cent of the persons admitted to mental hospitals ever fully recover. A somewhat larger proportion return to the community as improved but from 30 to 50 per cent of first admissions eventually die in a mental hospital.

A closer view of the effect of mental disease on mortality is seen by comparison of specific death rates among mental patients with those of the general population. Such comparison is shown by the accompanying table relating to death rates in New York State quoted from *Mortality Among Patients with Mental Disease* by Benjamin Malzberg, page 29.

Death rates among mental patients in the age groups from 15 to 29 years are more than 10 times as high as those among the general population; in the age groups from 30 to 49 years, more than 6 times as high; and in the age groups from 50 to 75, about 3 times as high.

It is evident that mental disease shortens life. The extent to which this is true in New York State is seen by the accompanying comparisons of expectations of life of mental patients with those of the general population at various ages.

At age 22, the expectation of life of a male patient in New York State in 1930 was 19 years as compared with 41.4 years for an average male in the general population; at age 32, the expectations for males in the two groups were 16.1 and 33.7 years, respectively. Like differences are noted for both sexes at all ages. It appears from these data that mental disease with its accompanying physical disorders reduces the average life expectancy of the afflicted by about one-half.

DEATH RATES BY AGE GROUPS AMONG PATIENTS WITH MENTAL DISEASE IN THE NEW YORK CIVIL STATE HOSPITALS, AND IN THE GENERAL POPULATION OF THE STATE OF NEW YORK, IN 1930

Age (years)	Average annual death rate among patients with mental disease (2)			Annual death rate in general population of New York State (3)		
	Males	Females	Total	Males	Females	Total
Under 15 (1)	20.6	12.1	17.5	1.6	1.2	1.4
15-19	58.2	52.3	55.8	2.5	2.1	2.3
20-24	45.7	55.8	49.8	3.3	3.1	3.2
25-29	36.5	50.5	42.6	3.9	3.5	3.7
30-34	38.2	42.6	40.4	5.0	3.9	4.5
35-39	44.3	41.2	42.7	6.5	4.7	5.6
40-44	51.7	45.1	48.4	9.0	6.6	7.8
45-49	59.7	48.5	54.1	13.1	9.5	11.4
50-54	72.8	55.4	63.4	19.4	13.4	16.5
55-59	89.8	68.4	78.0	27.0	20.3	23.6
60-64	135.3	90.4	110.2	38.8	30.5	34.6
65-69	172.0	120.9	143.3	53.6	44.3	48.8
70-74	256.8	171.5	207.1	76.6	65.6	70.8
75-79	339.5	239.3	280.0	112.4	102.1	106.8
80-84	418.1	321.0	357.5	167.8	148.0	156.3
85 and over	466.8	348.1	382.8	254.0	233.0	241.1

1. Among patients those under 15 are practically all from 10 to 14 years of age; the rate in the general population is therefore taken at ages 10 to 14.
2. Per 1,000 exposures.
3. Per 1,000 population.

EXPECTATION OF LIFE IN YEARS (1)

Age (years)	Patients with mental disease, 1930		Population of State of New York, 1920	
	Males	Females	Males	Females
22	19.02	18.18	41.40	42.98
27	17.96	18.28	37.54	39.19
32	16.10	17.67	33.74	35.44
37	14.21	16.26	29.98	31.57
42	12.40	14.61	26.25	27.63
47	10.67	12.86	22.59	23.79
52	8.92	10.92	19.08	20.11
57	7.17	8.97	15.83	16.68
62	5.46	7.16	12.88	13.52
67	3.98	5.53	10.22	10.71
72	2.84	4.15	7.94	8.40
77	2.21	3.02	6.00	6.48
82	1.75	2.21	4.38	4.85
87	1.48	1.60	3.07	3.50

(1) From *Life Tables for Patients with Mental Disease by* BENJAMIN MALZBERG, page 10.

5. Economic Loss Due to Mental Disease

Mental disease not only shortens life, but also reduces earning capacity and creates an enormous burden for society to bear. A mental patient, as long as his mental affliction persists, has practically no earning power. He must spend on the average from four to five years in a mental hospital. If death does not claim him, he may go out in the community as recovered or improved. Such event would indicate that a degree of working ability has been regained, but only in exceptional cases is complete restoration of efficiency experienced.

Such prolonged illness, in addition to being an irreparable loss to the afflicted individual and to society, involves great economic loss. An average man as a producing unit has a large money value. The following table, compiled from the book *The Money Value of a Man* by Dublin and Lotka, shows the value at various periods of life of a man whose maximum annual earning capacity is $2,000. Such a person at age 20 has a value of $23,850, at age 30, $24,450, and at age 40, $20,350. Thereafter his value declines rapidly.

Economic Value of a Man with Maximum Earning Capacity of $2,000, as Calculated by Drs. Dublin and Lotka

Age (years)	Value	Age (years)	Value
0	$7,000	40	$20,350
10	14,950	50	13,800
20	23,850	60	6,700
30	24,450	70	400

These data afford a basis for the calculation of the loss due to incapacity resulting from mental disease.* Careful estimates made from our New York data lead to the conclusion that when an individual suffers a mental breakdown and enters a mental hospital for the first time, his money value as a producing agent is on the average reduced by about 60 per cent. Males and females are found to suffer a like percentage of loss.

The other principal item of loss due to mental disease is the cost of care and treatment of the afflicted individuals. Such cost is

*See Chapter IV.

shared by the patient's family and the state or nation. In the United States each state maintains one or more state hospitals for mental patients, and bears the larger part of the expense of their maintenance. In New York State in 1936, the cost of hospital care and treatment of an average daily patient population of 67,000 amounted to about fifty million dollars. The loss in economic value suffered by the 13,220 first admissions to mental hospitals of that year was over one hundred million dollars. The total economic loss therefore was over one hundred and fifty million dollars. The average loss per family in the state was about forty dollars.

The economic loss in the United States as a whole on account of mental disease in 1936 was about one billion dollars. Such loss, great though it be, is small compared to the loss of health, the loss of mentality and the loss of life suffered by the afflicted individuals. These losses and those suffered by the families of patients are human values that cannot be expressed in financial terms.

6. The Relation of Mental Disease to Marriage and Reproduction

That mental disease is a deterrent to marriage and reproduction is self-evident. Naturally, nearly all those persons who develop mental disease while single do not later marry even though they may recover. Many relatives of mental patients are deterred from marriage for eugenic reasons. The numbers involved are significant but not large enough to affect seriously the general marriage rate.

Mental disease likewise lessens reproduction. Those persons who remain single because of mental disease have almost no children; those persons of child-bearing age who develop mental disease after marriage have few children after the onset of the disease.

A field study of 448 former female patients of the New York civil State hospitals was made in 1930 and 1931, 10 years after the patients had been discharged from the hospitals. Of these patients at the time of admission, 150 were single, 244 married, 35 widowed, 5 divorced and 14 separated. The children born alive to the several groups were as follows:

CHILDREN BORN TO FEMALE PATIENTS

Marital status	Female patients		Children	
	Before admission	After discharge	Born before admission	Born after discharge
Single	150	125	2	...
Married	244	224	613	118
Widowed	35	61	70	2
Divorced	5	7	3	0
Separated	14	31	24	2
Total	448	448	712	122

The 448 female patients, all of whom had reached the child-bearing age previous to admission, had a total of 834 children. The number of children per female patient was 1.86. Assuming half of the children to be females, the total female children born would be 417 and the gross reproduction rate would be 0.93. This rate is much lower than the average rate for females of the same age in the general population, and much too low for self-reproduction.

If like effects on reproduction obtain among the persons in the community who suffer with mild forms of mental disease, it would appear that mental disease is a factor of importance in reducing the general birth rate.

7. Mental Disease in Relation to Suicide and Crime

A person who becomes mentally ill thereby often loses the power of self-direction and self-control and the ability to inhibit or suppress his impulses. When he becomes deeply depressed, life may mean little or nothing to him, and the impulse to end it all may be welcomed and acted on when the occasion seems opportune.

The danger of suicide among mental patients is generally recognized by everyone charged with their care. In mental hospitals patients suspected of suicidal intent are specially safeguarded. The behavior of other patients is carefully watched for tendencies toward self-destruction. Were these precautions not taken, suicides among mental patients would be much more numerous than they now are.

It is believed that a large part of the suicides occurring in the community among the so-called normal population are due to mental disorder of some kind. However, the assumption that all persons who commit suicide were previously mentally ill is unwarranted. It is quite possible for a sane man to reach the conclusion that it is easier to kill himself than to face life's difficulties.

The magnitude of the problem of suicides is not fully revealed by statistics. It is believed to be much larger than the reported data would indicate. Likewise, the causes of suicides are not fully or correctly reported. For these reasons the part played by mental disease in this tragic phase of human behavior cannot be definitely measured, but is known to be very large.

That mental disorders of the lesser sort give rise to many forms of socially unacceptable behavior is everywhere recognized. They are among the prominent causes of dissension in the home, of inadequacy in work, of failure in business, and of maladjustment in social relations. These minor behavior disorders are endured by relatives and associates of the afflicted person, often for long periods. When the mental abnormality is not recognized or understood, the objectionable behavior may lead to quarreling, fighting or troublesome litigation.

When a mental disorder becomes so pronounced that reason is dethroned and the baser instincts gain mastery, the afflicted person becomes a social menace. If he is not given hospital care nor otherwise restrained, he may commit serious offenses such as reckless driving, arson, assault and homicide.

Perhaps the most dangerous types of mental patients are those who suffer from delusions of persecution. These patients feel that they have been unjustly treated, and often direct their animosity toward certain persons or groups who are entirely blameless. Such paranoid types are not commonly considered mentally diseased until they commit a crime or get into serious trouble. Even then their mental condition may be a matter of prolonged controversy.

Another troublesome type of mentally-disordered offender is the so-called psychopath. His antisocial behavior may take many different forms. He may wander from place to place as a hobo or tramp; he may become an alcoholic; he may indulge in sexual perversions; he may steal automobiles just for the pleasure of taking a ride; he may forge checks or engage in other fraudulent practices. If he is caught and given a jail sentence, he does not profit from the experience but resumes his criminal activities soon after discharge. His life thereafter is likely to be a series of jail terms interspersed with periods of freedom. Often the psychopathic individual becomes frankly psychotic and is committed to a mental hospital.

Persons with other forms of mental disease such as dementia præcox, manic-depressive psychosis, alcoholic psychosis, or general paresis frequently develop antisocial trends and commit serious offenses. In most of these cases the mental disease is evident, and the afflicted persons are committed either to a civil mental hospital or a hospital for the criminal insane.

As insane persons are usually not held responsible for their acts, the plea of insanity is frequently made in trials for murder. In doubtful cases long and bitter legal and psychiatric controversies are waged, generally at the expense and disgust of the general public. The difficulty experienced in drawing the line between responsibility and irresponsibility is evidenced by weighty and costly volumes of court decisions. Fortunately, many enlightened communities have found a way to settle, outside the court room, the question of the mental status of the accused.

The cost of crime in general reaches enormous proportions. The percentage of this great social burden that is properly chargeable to mental disease cannot be determined from data now available. Evidence at hand, however, indicates that such percentage is large, and that the total annual cost of crime due to mental disease in America alone reaches into the millions.

8. The Future of Mental Disease*

Mental disease throughout the world at present (1941) is an increasing rather than a decreasing social problem. The proportion of the population suffering from mental disease is constantly getting larger, and economic losses due to mental disease are continually mounting. The situation, however, is not without hope. Much has been learned concerning the causes and nature of the various abnormal mental conditions, and progress is being made in their treatment and prevention. If some great research worker like Pasteur should discover means of preventing arterio-

*See Chapter X.

sclerosis, dementia præcox and manic-depressive psychoses, the whole aspect of the problem would be changed. If important discoveries in this field are not made, mental disease, in the not distant future, will supersede physical disease as the paramount health problem. We can take courage from what has been accomplished in the field of physical disease, and we may confidently expect that by multiplying means of research and by diligently disseminating the recently acquired knowledge of mental hygiene, the burden of mental disease will be lessened for future generations.

REFERENCES

Brown, Frederick W.: A statistical survey of patients in hospitals for mental disease and institutions for feebleminded and epileptics in 32 countries. *The American Foundation for Mental Hygiene*, New York, 1930.

Malzberg, Benjamin: Expectation of mental disease in New York City, in 1930, *Mental Hygiene*, April, 1937.

Malzberg, Benjamin: Life tables for patients with mental disease, *Psychiatric Quarterly*, April, 1932.

Malzberg, Benjamin: Marital status in relation to the prevalence of mental disease, *Psychiatric Quarterly*, April, 1936.

Malzberg, Benjamin: Mortality among patients with mental disease, *State Hospitals Press*, 1934.

New York State Department of Mental Hygiene, Annual report, 1936.

Pollock, Horatio M.: Economic loss to New York State and the United States on account of mental disease, 1931, *Mental Hygiene*, April, 1932.

Pollock,Horatio M., and Benjamin Malzberg: Expectation of mental disease, *Psychiatric Quarterly*, October, 1928.

Pollock, Horatio M.: The future of mental disease from a statistical viewpoint, *American Journal of Psychiatry*, January, 1924.

U. S. Bureau of Census, Patients in all hospitals for mental disease, 1935.

U. S. Bureau of Census, Patients in hospitals for mental disease, 1923.

CHAPTER II

The Expectation of Mental Disease*

The probability of developing a mental disorder, as measured by rates of first admissions, is a function of age. The probability is exceedingly small in childhood, but rises thereafter with advancing age, the probability being a maximum in old age. We may ask, however, what is the probability of developing a mental disorder not at a specified age, but in the course of a generation. The question was first raised in this form by Dr. Thomas W. Salmon. He attempted to find an answer by comparing deaths in a single year in New York State in hospitals for mental disease with those in the general population. He found that in a given year 1-22 of the deaths reported to the New York State Health Department occurred in hospitals for mental patients. Comparing deaths in such hospitals with admissions, he found that the latter were approximately twice as great as the former. He concluded from these data that about one out of every ten or eleven persons became mentally ill in the course of a generation. The estimate was made from data drawn from several generations and proved much too high.

A preliminary combined mortality and mental disease table prepared at the time of Dr. Salmon's inquiry in the statistical bureau of the New York State Hospital Commission from crude data gave the proportion of those becoming mentally ill in the course of a generation as approximately 1 in 25.

The present analysis is an attempt to show more definitely the expectation of mental disease in New York State not only at birth but at every age of life. The life table method of analysis has been used and the data have been segregated by sex and nativity. So far as known this is the first attempt to produce standard, combined life and mental disease tables.

The data with respect to mental disease were derived from individual statistical schedules of first admissions prepared in the State hospitals and licensed institutions for mental disease in New York State, and sent regularly to the statistical bureau of the Department of Mental Hygiene.

*Dr. Benjamin Malzberg collaborated with the author in the preparation of this chapter.

Cases of mental disease too mild to require admission to a hospital were not included in the analysis.

In order to secure an adequate number of cases for detailed analysis the first admissions of 1919, 1920 and 1921 were taken, comprising a total of 21,997 cases. These were subdivided as follows: native males, 6,362; native females, 5,697; foreign-born males, 5,373; foreign-born females, 4,565. Each nativity group was classified by age and sex and the average annual number of first admissions of each class was computed.

Corresponding data for the general population of the State of New York were taken from the U. S. Census of 1920 and were adjusted to read as of July 1, 1920. As is always to be expected in such data, there was great irregularity in the age distribution of the patients and of the general population and it was consequently necessary to smooth the data before beginning the analysis. Both the hospital admissions and the general population were grouped into quinquennial age periods. The subsequent smoothing and interpolations were made by applying the method of osculatory interpolation. From the smoothed data the probability of mental disease at each age was obtained by the usual formula, that is $s_x = \frac{2i_x}{2l_{x+\frac{1}{2}} + i_x}$ where s_x represents the probability of mental disease at exact age x, i_x, the number becoming mental patients during the xth year, and $l_{x+\frac{1}{2}}$ the total population at age $(x+\frac{1}{2})$. Good results were obtained for almost the entire range of the table. There were, however, so few cases under 13 years of age that it was necessary to assume that the incidence of mental disease began at that age. This is in fact a safe assumption, as data carefully gathered for many years show that there are very few first admissions under 15 years of age, the exceptions being a small number of children suffering from epidemic encephalitis. There was corresponding difficulty at the other end of the table, as there were too few cases past 90 years of age to yield adequate rates. Consequently, the data, where necessary, were completed by extrapolating the rates graphically on the assumption of a parabolic distribution. As will be shown in the tables, there are so few mentally ill individuals to be expected at these ages that it would require an error in the corresponding rates of mental disease amounting to an exceedingly high order to cause any significant difference in the resulting probabilities.

As noted above, the rates of mental disease were computed for individual years, for each sex, under the categories of native and foreign-born. The nativity groups were then combined and two additional tables were constructed representing total males and females in the State of New York.

In carrying out the analysis it was necessary to make use of rates of mortality in conjunction with the probabilities of mental disease. Because of the fact that no complete life tables were available that included exactly the same elements as those utilized in the present analysis, it was necessary to make certain assumptions. There was no complete life table for the State of New York for 1920 for all males or for all females. It was therefore necessary to use tables for the U. S. Registration States, and these were kindly furnished by Dr. Louis I. Dublin, statistician of the Metropolitan Life Insurance Company, in whose statistical bureau the abridged Foudray 1920 table was completed for all intervening years. In the remaining cases it was possible to use data for the State of New York. These consist of life tables prepared in the Division of Vital Statistics in the New York State Department of Health for the following groups: Native males, native females, foreign-born males and foreign-born females. These tables, however, all began with age 20, due to the fact that in the foreign-born groups there were too few individuals at the earlier ages to permit the calculation of accurate mortality rates. In order to make the life tables directly comparable, those with respect to nativity were therefore begun at age 20. Since, for the purpose of the present investigation, mortality rates were needed for each year, they were supplied from birth to the 20th year on the following assumptions: In the case of the native group, it was assumed that the ratio of the mortality rates at each year under 20 in 1920 to the corresponding rates in 1910, as given by Glover, was equal to the ratio of the mortality rates in 1920 at each age under 20, as given by Dr. Dublin for total whites in the U. S. Registration area, to the rates in the U. S. Registration area in 1910, as given by Glover. In the case of the foreign-born females, such assumptions gave discordant results and it was thought better, therefore, to apply the Dublin values for total white females for ages 0 to 20. Similarly in the case of the foreign-born males, the mortality rates from birth through the fifth year were assumed to be the same as given by Dublin for the native males. It is true that this introduces an element of uncertainty, but the resultant error, if any, will be a slight underestimate rather than an overestimate as the mortality rates for the foreign-born actually exceed those for the native population. However, the final error cannot be great because of the fact that the essential data relating to the number of the mentally ill do not begin until age 13, and the subsequent rates up to age 20, where the rates of mortality and mental disease refer to the same nativity groups, are too low to cause any significant statistical errors.

The subsequent analysis was made in the following manner. The total population alive and sane at the exact age x was multiplied by the corresponding value of s_x to obtain the number, i_x, becoming mentally ill in that age interval. If i_x is then deducted from l_x, the remainder will represent the number alive at age x who did not become mentally ill during that year; this new total, multiplied by q_x, the life table rate of mortality, gives the number of the latter group who will die in the xth year. Deducting these deaths gives the population alive and sane at exact age x+1. This procedure is followed for each age until the entire population has disappeared. The method may be more clearly understood by referring to Table 3, showing the probability of mental disease among total males in the State of New York in 1920. This begins with a population of 100,000 at birth. It will be noticed that there are no mental cases until the 13th year is attained. Consequently up to that year, each yearly population need only be multiplied by the rate of mortality and the corresponding deduction made to obtain the population at the succeeding age level which has remained both alive and mentally well. At age 13, there is of the original group a total of 86,388 living and sane individuals. Multiplying this total by 5.6, the rate of mental disease per 100,000 population at age 13, there results an expectation of 5 cases of mental disease. Deducting these from 86,388, there is obtained the population alive at exact age 13, who did not become mentally diseased in the 13th year. Multiplying this number, 86,383, by the rate of mortality per thousand, 2.4, gives the expected number of deaths, 207, which when deducted from 86,383 gives 86,176 as the number of white males remaining alive and sane at exact age 14 out of a population of 100,000 at birth. This procedure thus gives the number becoming mentally ill in each age interval until the entire population has disappeared.

Beginning then with the last year to provide any cases of mental disease, proceed to add cumulatively back to birth. The cumulative total at each age tells how many individuals out of those alive and sane at that age became mentally diseased before death. Dividing the cumulative total at any age by the population alive and sane at that age gives the expectation of mental disease at such age. Each expectation was reduced to the basis of 100. Thus, in the case of the total males the expectation at birth is that 4.7 per 100 will become mentally diseased before death.

Table 1 is a summarized statement of the expectations of mental disease in the several groups, beginning with birth. It should be noted that the expectation at birth of the males exceeded that of the females. In the total groups the expectations at birth were 4.7 per 100 for males and 4.4 for females. These increased to maxima at age 15 of 5.5 for males and of 5.1 for females. In succeeding years there was a continuous decrease. As the cumulative total of the mentally ill was the same from birth to the 13th year, the increased expectancy up to the latter year can be entirely accounted for by the decreasing function l_x which furnishes the denominator in the expression for the expectation of mental disease.

If, now, the first admissions are analyzed according to nativity, it is seen that the expectation of mental disease at birth was higher among the foreign-born than among the natives. Among males, the expectation was 5.4 per cent for foreign-born and 4.3 for natives. Among females the corresponding expectations were 5.2

and 4.0 per cent. In each nativity group there was an increase in the expectation of mental disease until approximately the 14th year, after which the expectations decreased steadily to minima in old age.

TABLE 1. NUMBER BECOMING MENTALLY ILL DURING REMAINDER OF LIFE OF 100 ALIVE AND SANE AT SPECIFIED AGE, BY NATIVITY AND SEX

Exact age in years	Total		Native		Foreign-born	
	Male	Female	Male	Female	Male	Female
0	4.7	4.4	4.3	4.0	5.4	5.2
5	5.4	5.0	4.9	4.4	6.1	5.8
10	5.4	5.1	5.0	4.4	6.2	5.8
15	5.5	5.1	5.0	4.5	6.2	5.9
20	5.3	5.0	4.9	4.4	5.8	5.7
25	5.0	4.9	4.6	4.3	5.3	5.4
30	4.7	4.6	4.3	4.1	4.9	5.1
35	4.4	4.4	4.0	3.8	4.4	4.7
40	4.0	4.1	3.7	3.5	4.0	4.3
45	3.7	3.8	3.4	3.2	3.6	4.0
50	3.4	3.4	3.1	2.9	3.3	3.6
55	3.1	3.1	2.8	2.6	3.0	3.3
60	2.8	2.9	2.6	2.4	2.8	3.1
65	2.6	2.6	2.4	2.2	2.5	2.9
70	2.3	2.4	2.1	2.0	2.3	2.7
75	2.0	2.2	1.8	1.9	2.1	2.4
80	1.8	2.0	1.5	1.7	1.9	2.2
85	1.5	1.6	1.2	1.4	1.7	1.9
90	1.2	1.3	1.0	1.2	1.4	1.7
95	1.0	1.0	0.7	1.0	0.9	1.4

Table 2 summarizes the rates of first admissions. There was a gradual increase in the rates from adolescence to old age, with the exception of a slight decrease among males in the fourth and fifth decades of life. The native population showed similar trends. The rates for the foreign-born males did not show the same regularity, however. This resulted in all probability from the high rate of dementia præcox among the younger foreign-born males. After 50 years of age, however, a steady increase was clearly evidenced. The rates for foreign-born females were lower than those for foreign-born males up to the forty-fifth year, but thereafter the rates for males were lower. In the native group no such marked differences were found in the rates for the two sexes in the early ages. The explanation may, perhaps, be found in the greater difficulty that the older foreign-born female finds in adjusting herself to different patterns of behavior and culture.

TABLE 2. SUMMARY OF AVERAGE ANNUAL RATES OF FIRST ADMISSIONS PER 100,000 GENERAL POPULATION TO ALL HOSPITALS FOR MENTAL DISEASES IN NEW YORK, 1919-1921 INCLUSIVE, BY AGE, NATIVITY AND SEX

Exact age in years	Total		Native		Foreign-born	
	Male	Female	Male	Female	Male	Female
0	....	....	....	....	....	....
5	....	....	....	....	....	....
10	....	....	....	....	....	....
15	34.8	24.4	29.2	18.2	86.1	51.7
20	78.1	47.5	68.4	42.2	131.8	71.3
25	94.6	70.0	83.4	61.9	129.2	94.1
30	101.6	86.6	91.4	76.9	123.4	106.8
35	106.6	91.4	98.1	85.1	124.0	107.5
40	107.7	94.0	102.1	92.5	123.4	108.5
45	102.2	99.8	96.7	94.3	114.2	117.1
50	98.6	105.6	94.0	95.7	108.9	122.0
55	106.4	108.4	101.2	98.2	116.0	119.9
60	122.1	110.5	117.1	101.2	131.8	124.8
65	148.5	134.7	142.7	112.3	160.3	162.7
70	190.1	166.7	183.9	136.0	203.4	217.0
75	219.7	213.8	215.0	180.2	239.0	268.9
80	260.5	279.9	245.1	234.2	291.0	353.4
85	314.0	324.5	275.0	285.5	370.5	414.0
90	345.0	347.0	306.1	343.0	433.0	482.0
95	388.5	412.5	337.0	427.0	511.0	598.0

Complete data for each year of life are shown in Tables 3-8.

Charts 1 and 2 show comparative curves of expectation of mental disease among the several age and sex groups covering the entire life span. Chart 1 gives a graphic comparison of the expectation of mental disease among males and females. The rates among males were the higher up to age 34. From age 34 to age 65 the rates for the two sexes were nearly equal, those of the females being slightly in excess. After age 65 the higher rates of the females were more marked.

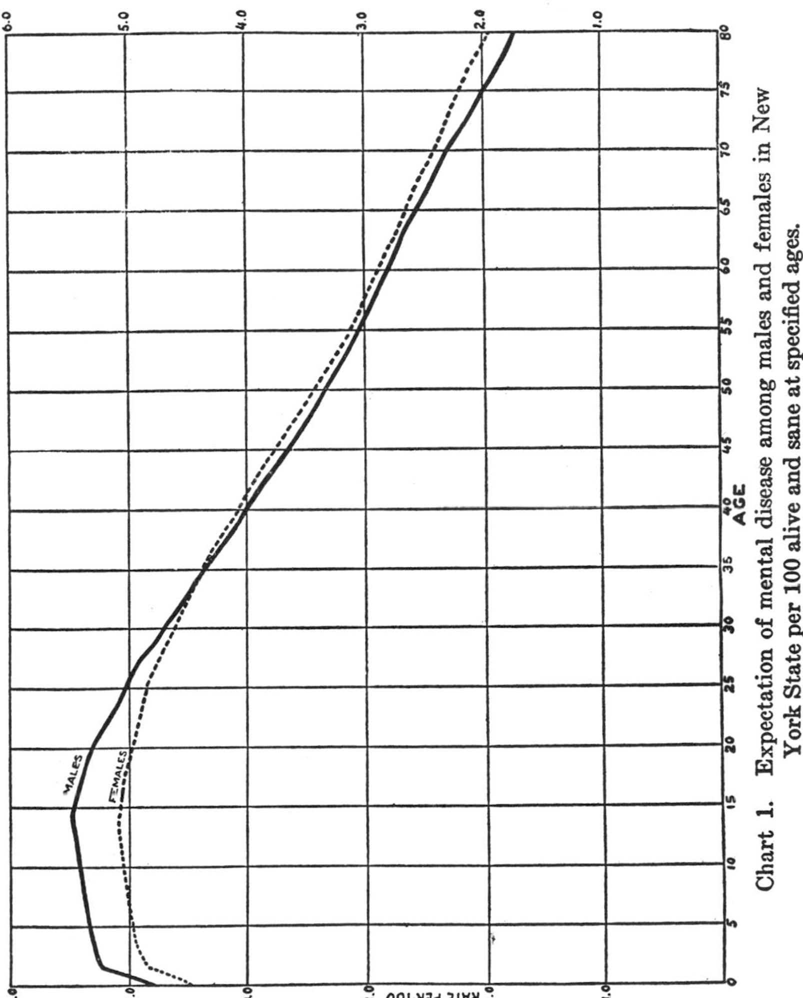

Chart 1. Expectation of mental disease among males and females in New York State per 100 alive and sane at specified ages.

Chart 2 compares the expectation of mental disease by sex throughout life among the native and foreign-born. The expectation of mental disease began among the native males with 4.3 per cent at birth, and rose to a maximum of 5.0 from the 10th to the 17th year. It then decreased regularly to the end of the life span. The expectation of the native females, beginning with 4.0 per cent at birth rose to a maximum of 4.5 from the 12th to the 16th year, and decreased regularly thereafter. The expectation of the males was in excess of that of the females until the 74th year.

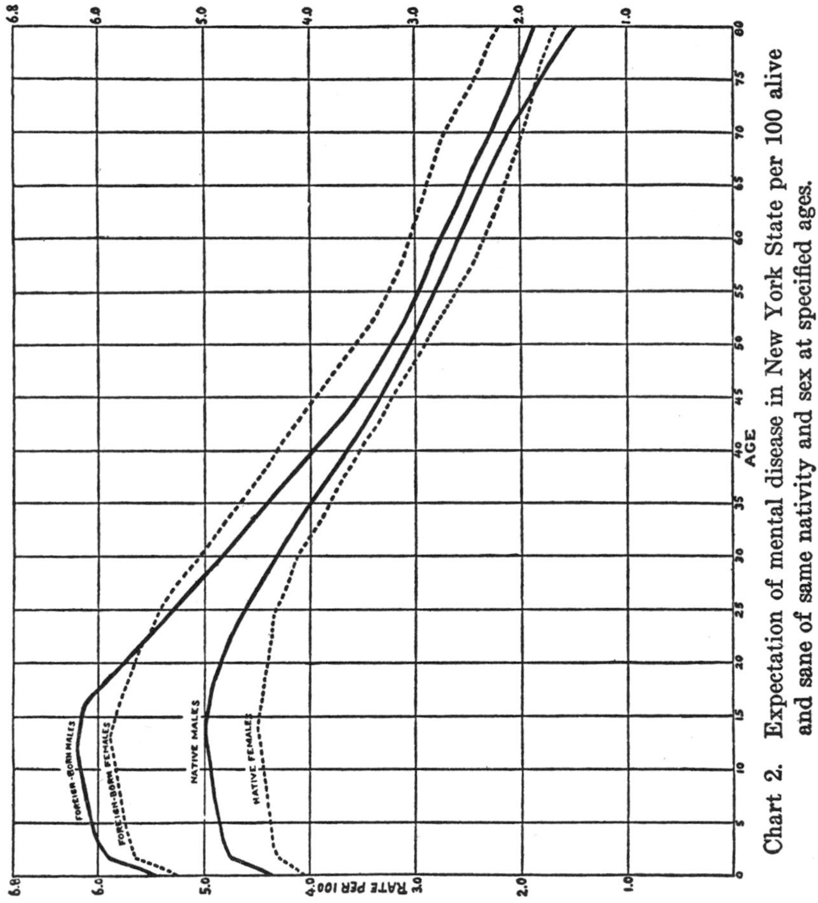

Chart 2. Expectation of mental disease in New York State per 100 alive and sane of same nativity and sex at specified ages.

In the case of the foreign-born, the expectation of mental disease increased among males from 5.4 per cent at birth to a maximum of 6.2 from the 9th to the 15th year, and decreased thereafter. The expectation of the foreign-born females was lower than that of the males, beginning with 5.2 per cent at birth and rising to a maximum of 5.9 from the 11th to the 15th year; beyond the 25th year the expectation of the females exceeded that of the males.

Charts 3 and 4 show rates of incidence of serious mental disease per 100,000 of population of same age, sex and nativity. As previously mentioned, the rates were based upon the average annual first admissions to all institutions for mental disease in New York State during the fiscal years ended June 30, 1919, 1920 and 1921. The population data were derived from the Federal Census of New York State of 1920. Both sets of data were smoothed before the rates were computed.

Chart 3 compares rates of mental disease among males and females from 13 to 80 years of age. It will be noted that the males had the higher rates from age 14 to age 45 and from age 56 to age 76. The rates of both sexes increased with advancing age, except for a slight reduction among the males from age 42 to age 56.

Chart 4 compares rates of mental disease by sex among the native and foreign-born populations of the State. The rates of the native groups were lower than those of the corresponding foreign-born groups at every age. In both nativity groups the males had higher rates than the females, except during the involutional and advanced age periods. These comparative rates are relatively similar to those shown by the Federal census report of "Patients in Hospitals for Mental Disease, 1923" (Page 32), although the rates for New York are higher than those shown for the country as a whole.

The data of this study emphasize the seriousness of the problem of mental disease. It appears that approximately 4.5 per cent of the persons born in the State of New York may, under existing conditions, be expected to succumb to mental disease of one form or another, and become patients in the hospitals for mental disease. In other words, on the average, approximately 1 person out of 22 becomes a patient in a hospital for mental disease during the life time of a generation. In the several groups shown in the tables the ratios of those becoming patients to the whole population group are as follows: All males, 1 to 21.3; all females, 1 to 22.7; native males, 1 to 23.3; native females, 1 to 25.0; foreign-born males, 1 to 18.5; foreign-born females, 1 to 19.2.

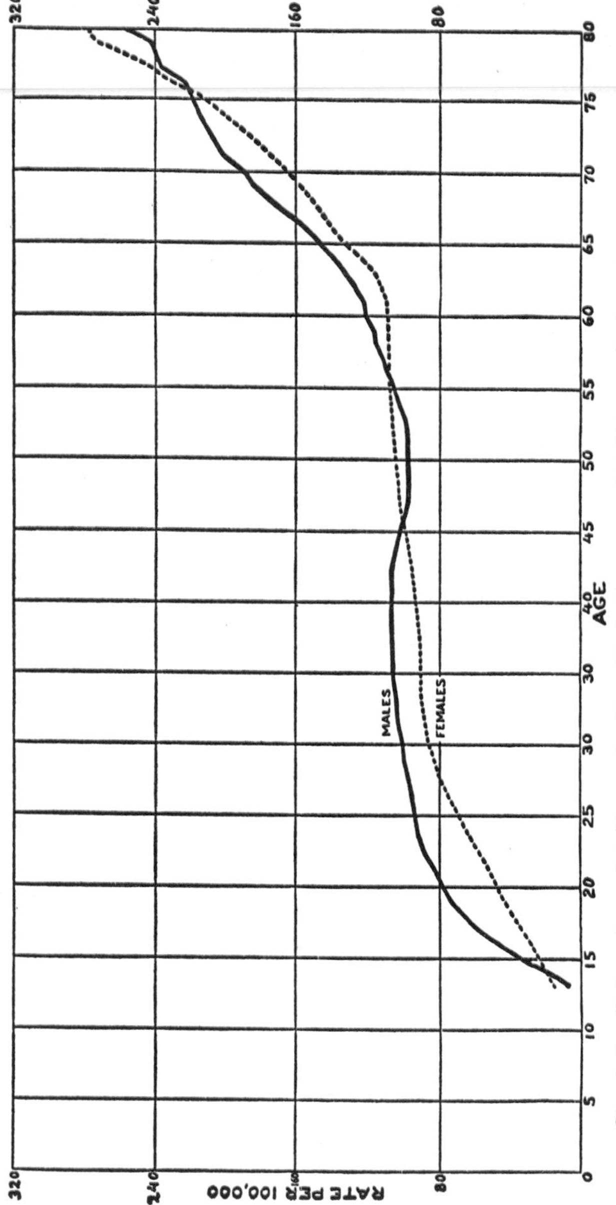

Chart 3. Rates of mental disease in New York State per 100,000 population of same age and sex.

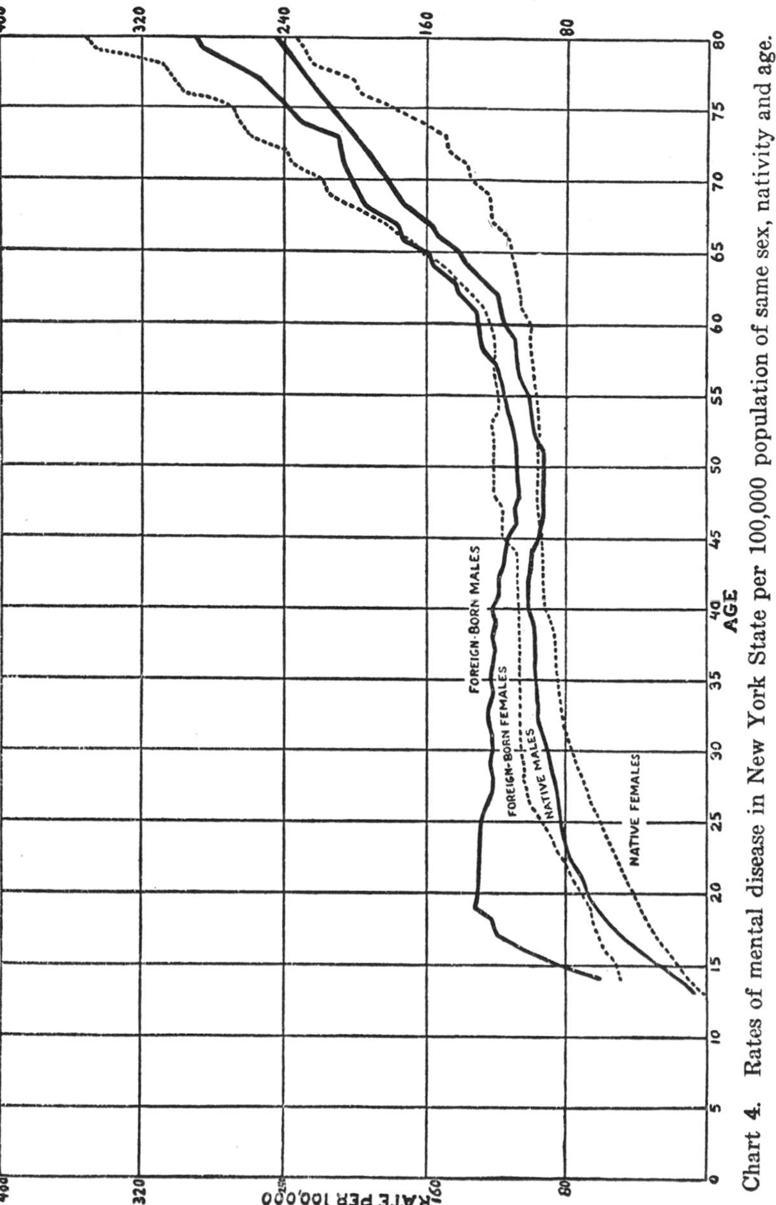

Chart 4. Rates of mental disease in New York State per 100,000 population of same sex, nativity and age.

From the data presented in the tables similar ratios may be computed for all of the groups at any age of life. Given the age and nativity composition of any group of persons, the proportion that will probably develop serious mental disease may be determined by applying the appropriate expectation rates as given in the tables. The following tabulation furnishes simple illustrations.

PROBABLE NUMBER AMONG CERTAIN SOCIAL GROUPS WHO WILL DEVELOP SERIOUS MENTAL DISEASE AND BECOME PATIENTS IN A HOSPITAL FOR MENTAL DISEASE*

	Probable cases of mental disease
Among 117,000 male children born in New York State in 1927	5,000
Among 110,000 female children born in New York State in 1927	4,400
Among 1,030,000 boys in public schools of New York State in 1927	51,500
Among 990,000 girls in public schools in New York State in 1927	44,000
Among 194,000 male immigrants to the United States in year ended June 30, 1927	10,000
Among 141,000 female immigrants to the United States in year ended June 30, 1927	7,300
Among 3,500,000 World War veterans with average age of 35 years	154,000

*Round numbers are used, as most of the data given are approximations.

In presenting these results it is not desired to leave the impression that mental disease is a fatalistic matter; that it is as certain as old age or death. Under present conditions, however, mental disease occurs among the general population with striking regularity and it seems probable that the rate of incidence will not greatly change until the principles of mental hygiene are better known and more widely adopted.

TABLE 3. EXPECTATION OF MENTAL DISEASE AMONG MALES IN NEW YORK STATE, 1920

Age interval, years	Of 100,000 persons born alive		Rate of mental disease per 100,000	Rate of mortality per 1,000	Expectation of mental disease
Period of life-time between two exact ages	Number alive and sane at beginning of age interval	Number becoming mentally ill in age interval	Number becoming mentally ill during age interval among 100,000 alive and sane at beginning of age interval	Number dying in age interval per 1,000 alive at beginning of interval and remaining sane during interval	Number becoming mentally ill during remainder of life of 100 alive and sane at beginning of age interval
x to $x+1$	l_x	i_x	$100{,}000\,s_x$	$1{,}000\,q_x$	$t_x = \frac{100 \Sigma i_x}{l_x}$
0-1	100,000	...	...	84.3	4.7
1-2	91,570	...	...	17.6	5.2
2-3	89,958	...	...	8.5	5.3
3-4	89,193	...	...	5.9	5.3
4-5	88,667	...	...	4.6	5.3
5-6	88,259	...	...	3.9	5.4
6-7	87,915	...	...	3.4	5.4
7-8	87,616	...	...	3.0	5.4
8-9	87,353	...	...	2.5	5.4
9-10	87,135	...	...	2.2	5.4
10-11	86,943	...	...	2.1	5.4
11-12	86,760	...	...	2.1	5.4
12-13	86,578	...	...	2.2	5.4
13-14	86,388	5	5.6	2.4	5.4
14-15	86,176	17	19.3	2.7	5.4
15-16	85,943	30	34.8	3.2	5.4
16-17	85,638	41	47.3	3.6	5.4
17-18	85,289	50	58.7	3.9	5.4
18-19	84,907	56	66.5	4.2	5.4
19-20	84,495	63	74.2	4.4	5.4
20-21	84,060	66	78.1	4.6	5.3
21-22	83,608	69	82.7	4.8	5.3
22-23	83,138	73	87.8	5.0	5.2
23-24	82,650	75	91.0	5.1	5.1
24-25	82,154	76	93.0	5.3	5.1
25-26	81,643	77	94.6	5.4	5.0
26-27	81,126	77	95.4	5.6	5.0
27-28	80,595	78	96.9	5.8	4.9
28-29	80,050	79	98.3	6.0	4.8
29-30	79,491	80	100.2	6.2	4.8
30-31	78,919	80	101.6	6.5	4.7
31-32	78,327	81	103.3	6.7	4.6
32-33	77,722	81	104.3	6.9	4.6
33-34	77,105	82	105.8	7.0	4.5
34-35	76,484	81	106.0	7.2	4.4
35-36	75,853	81	106.6	7.3	4.4

TABLE 3. EXPECTATION OF MENTAL DISEASE AMONG MALES IN NEW YORK STATE, 1920—(*Continued*)

Age interval, years	Of 100,000 persons born alive		Rate of mental disease per 100,000	Rate of mortality per 1,000	Expectation of mental disease
Period of lifetime between two exact ages	Number alive and sane at beginning of age interval	Number becoming mentally ill in age interval	Number becoming mentally ill during age interval among 100,000 alive and sane at beginning of age interval	Number dying in age interval per 1,000 alive at beginning of interval and remaining sane during interval	Number becoming mentally ill during remainder of life of 100 alive and sane at beginning of age interval
x to $x+1$	l_x	i_x	$100{,}000\, s_x$	$1{,}000\, q_x$	$\frac{t_x = \sum_x^{100} i_x}{l_x}$
36-37	75,219	81	107.2	7.4	4.3
37-38	74,582	80	107.3	7.6	4.2
38-39	73,936	80	107.6	7.8	4.1
39-40	73,280	79	108.0	8.0	4.1
40-41	72,614	78	107.7	8.2	4.0
41-42	71,941	77	107.5	8.4	3.9
42-43	71,260	77	107.4	8.7	3.9
43-44	70,564	75	106.1	8.9	3.8
44-45	69,862	73	104.9	9.2	3.7
45-46	69,147	71	102.2	9.5	3.7
46-47	68,420	69	101.0	9.9	3.6
47-48	67,674	67	99.7	10.4	3.5
48-49	66,904	66	99.0	10.9	3.4
49-50	66,109	65	98.4	11.5	3.4
50-51	65,284	64	98.6	12.2	3.4
51-52	64,424	64	99.0	12.9	3.3
52-53	63,530	63	99.6	13.8	3.2
53-54	62,591	63	100.6	14.9	3.2
54-55	61,596	64	104.1	16.1	3.1
55-56	60,541	64	106.4	17.4	3.1
56-57	59,425	65	110.2	18.8	3.0
57-58	58,244	65	112.1	20.3	3.0
58-59	56,998	66	116.2	21.7	2.9
59-60	55,697	66	117.8	23.1	2.9
60-61	54,346	66	122.1	24.6	2.8
61-62	52,945	65	123.7	26.3	2.8
62-63	51,489	66	128.7	28.4	2.7
63-64	49,963	67	134.5	30.7	2.7
64-65	48,364	68	141.1	33.4	2.7
65-66	46,683	69	148.5	36.4	2.6
66-67	44,917	70	156.7	39.6	2.5
67-68	43,071	71	165.5	43.1	2.5
68-69	41,147	71	174.9	46.9	2.4
69-70	39,149	73	185.2	51.1	2.4
70-71	37,079	70	190.1	55.5	2.3
71-72	34,955	71	201.9	60.3	2.3

TABLE 3. EXPECTATION OF MENTAL DISEASE AMONG MALES IN NEW YORK STATE, 1920—(*Continued*)

Age interval, years	Of 100,000 persons born alive		Rate of mental disease per 100,000	Rate of mortality per 1,000	Expectation of mental disease
Period of lifetime between two exact ages	Number alive and sane at beginning of age interval	Number becoming mentally ill in age interval	Number becoming mentally ill during age interval among 100,000 alive and sane at beginning of age interval	Number dying in age interval per 1,000 alive at beginning of interval and remaining sane during interval	Number becoming mentally ill during remainder of life of 100 alive and sane at beginning of age interval
x to $x+1$	l_x	i_x	$100,000\, s_x$	$1,000\, q_x$	$t_x = \frac{\sum_x^{100} i_x}{l_x}$
72-73	32,780	68	207.3	65.4	2.2
73-74	30,573	65	212.2	70.8	2.1
74-75	28,348	61	215.9	76.4	2.1
75-76	26,126	57	219.7	82.4	2.0
76-77	23,921	53	222.3	89.0	2.0
77-78	21,744	52	237.4	96.4	1.9
78-79	19,601	47	240.1	104.8	1.8
79-80	17,505	42	241.6	114.2	1.8
80-81	15,469	40	260.5	124.4	1.8
81-82	13,510	38	282.6	135.2	1.7
82-83	11,651	36	307.5	146.0	1.7
83-84	9,919	31	309.1	156.8	1.6
84-85	8,334	26	311.5	167.8	1.5
85-86	6,914	22	314.0	179.3	1.5
86-87	5,656	18	316.2	191.2	1.4
87-88	4,560	15	318.5	204.0	1.4
88-89	3,618	12	327.5	217.8	1.3
89-90	2,821	9	336.0	232.6	1.2
90-91	2,158	7	345.0	248.2	1.2
91-92	1,617	6	353.6	264.0	1.2
92-93	1,186	4	362.5	279.7	1.1
93-94	851	3	371.0	294.6	1.1
94-95	598	2	379.5	308.7	1.0
95-96	412	2	388.5	323.0	1.0
96-97	278	1	397.0	338.5	0.7
97-98	183	1	406.0	356.5	0.5
98-99	117	...	414.5	377.5	...
99-100	73	...	...	401.2	...
100-101	44	...	...	427.1	...
101-102	25	...	...	454.8	...
102-103	14	...	...	483.7	...
103-104	7	...	...	...	...
104-105	4	...	...	...	...
105-106	1	...	...	...	...
106-107	1	...	...	...	...
107-108	...	...	...	...	...

TABLE 4. EXPECTATION OF MENTAL DISEASE AMONG FEMALES IN NEW YORK STATE, 1920

Age interval, years	Of 100,000 persons born alive		Rate of mental disease per 100,000	Rate of mortality per 1,000	Expectation of mental disease
Period of lifetime between two exact ages	Number alive and sane at beginning of age interval	Number becoming mentally ill in age interval	Number becoming mentally ill during age interval among 100,000 alive and sane at beginning of age interval	Number dying in age interval per 1,000 alive at beginning of interval and remaining sane during interval	Number becoming mentally ill during remainder of life of 100 alive and sane at beginning of age interval
x to $x + 1$	l_x	i_x	$100{,}000\, s_x$	$1{,}000\, q_x$	$t_x = \frac{\sum_x^{100} i_x}{l_x}$
0-1	100,000	...	...	67.3	4.4
1-2	93,270	...	...	15.8	4.8
2-3	91,796	...	...	7.7	4.9
3-4	91,089	...	...	5.6	4.9
4-5	90,579	...	...	4.1	5.0
5-6	90,208	...	...	3.6	5.0
6-7	89,883	...	...	3.1	5.0
7-8	89,604	...	...	2.6	5.0
8-9	89,371	...	...	2.2	5.0
9-10	89,174	...	...	1.9	5.0
10-11	89,005	...	...	1.8	5.1
11-12	88,845	...	...	1.8	5.1
12-13	88,685	...	...	1.9	5.1
13-14	88,516	13	15.2	2.1	5.1
14-15	88,317	17	19.6	2.3	5.1
15-16	88,097	21	24.4	2.7	5.1
16-17	87,838	25	28.7	3.1	5.1
17-18	87,541	30	34.1	3.5	5.1
18-19	87,205	35	39.6	3.8	5.0
19-20	86,839	38	44.1	4.3	5.0
20-21	86,428	41	47.5	4.7	5.0
21-22	85,981	45	51.9	5.1	5.0
22-23	85,498	48	56.1	5.4	4.9
23-24	84,989	52	61.0	5.7	4.9
24-25	84,453	55	65.6	6.0	4.9
25-26	83,892	59	70.0	6.2	4.9
26-27	83,313	62	74.4	6.4	4.8
27-28	82,718	65	78.2	6.5	4.8
28-29	82,116	67	81.3	6.7	4.7
29-30	81,499	68	83.1	6.8	4.7
30-31	80,877	70	86.6	6.9	4.6
31-32	80,249	70	87.7	6.9	4.6
32-33	79,626	71	89.0	7.0	4.5
33-34	78,998	72	90.9	7.0	4.4
34-35	78,374	71	91.1	7.0	4.4
35-36	77,755	71	91.4	7.0	4.4

TABLE 4. EXPECTATION OF MENTAL DISEASE AMONG FEMALES IN NEW YORK STATE, 1920—(*Continued*)

Age interval, years	Of 100,000 persons born alive		Rate of mental disease per 100,000	Rate of mortality per 1,000	Expectation of mental disease
Period of life-time between two exact ages	Number alive and sane at beginning of age interval	Number becoming mentally ill in age interval	Number becoming mentally ill during age interval among 100,000 alive and sane at beginning of age interval	Number dying in age interval per 1,000 alive at beginning of interval and remaining sane during interval	Number becoming mentally ill during remainder of life of 100 alive and sane at beginning of age interval
x to $x+1$	l_x	i_x	$100{,}000\, s_x$	$1{,}000\, q_x$	$t_x = \frac{100 \sum i_x}{l_x}$
36-37	77,140	71	91.6	7.0	4.3
37-38	76,530	70	91.8	7.0	4.3
38-39	75,925	70	92.1	7.1	4.2
39-40	75,316	70	93.1	7.1	4.1
40-41	74,712	70	94.0	7.2	4.1
41-42	74,105	70	95.0	7.4	4.0
42-43	73,487	71	96.1	7.6	4.0
43-44	72,858	71	97.2	7.8	3.9
44-45	72,219	71	98.4	8.1	3.8
45-46	71,564	71	99.8	8.5	3.8
46-47	70,885	72	101.2	8.9	3.7
47-48	70,183	72	102.7	9.3	3.6
48-49	69,459	72	103.6	9.8	3.6
49-50	68,707	72	104.5	10.3	3.5
50-51	67,928	72	105.6	10.9	3.4
51-52	67,116	72	106.7	11.6	3.4
52-53	66,266	71	107.1	12.4	3.3
53-54	65,374	70	107.8	13.3	3.2
54-55	64,435	70	108.1	14.3	3.2
55-56	63,445	69	108.4	15.4	3.1
56-57	62,400	68	108.9	16.6	3.1
57-58	61,297	67	109.3	17.9	3.0
58-59	60,134	66	109.6	19.1	3.0
59-60	58,921	65	110.1	20.4	2.9
60-61	57,655	64	110.5	21.8	2.9
61-62	56,336	62	110.6	23.4	2.8
62-63	54,957	63	114.0	25.3	2.8
63-64	53,505	63	117.8	27.5	2.7
64-65	51,972	65	125.8	30.1	2.7
65-66	50,345	68	134.7	33.0	2.6
66-67	48,618	68	140.4	36.1	2.6
67-68	46,797	69	146.4	39.4	2.6
68-69	44,887	69	152.8	42.9	2.5
69-70	42,895	68	159.5	46.7	2.4
70-71	40,827	68	166.7	50.9	2.4
71-72	38,684	68	174.6	55.3	2.4

TABLE 4. EXPECTATION OF MENTAL DISEASE AMONG FEMALES IN NEW YORK STATE, 1920—(*Continued*)

Age interval, years	Of 100,000 persons born alive		Rate of mental disease per 100,000	Rate of mortality per 1,000	Expectation of mental disease
Period of life-time between two exact ages	Number alive and sane at beginning of age interval	Number becoming mentally ill in age interval	Number becoming mentally ill during age interval among 100,000 alive and sane at beginning of age interval	Number dying in age interval per 1,000 alive at beginning of interval and remaining sane during interval	Number becoming mentally ill during remainder of life of 100 alive and sane at beginning of age interval
x to $x+1$	l_x	i_x	$100{,}000\, s_x$	$1{,}000\, q_x$	$t_x = \frac{\sum^{100}_x i_x}{l_x}$
72-73	36,481	67	183.2	60.1	2.3
73-74	34,226	66	192.5	65.2	2.3
74-75	31,933	65	202.7	70.7	2.3
75-76	29,615	63	213.8	76.6	2.2
76-77	27,288	62	226.1	83.1	2.2
77-78	24,964	60	240.1	90.1	2.1
78-79	22,660	58	256.1	97.9	2.1
79-80	20,389	56	274.4	106.6	2.0
80-81	18,166	51	279.9	116.0	2.0
81-82	16,014	48	302.0	125.8	1.9
82-83	13,957	43	306.8	135.8	1.8
83-84	12,024	40	332.2	145.9	1.8
84-85	10,236	34	332.9	156.2	1.7
85-86	8,608	29	334.5	167.0	1.6
86-87	7,146	24	336.1	178.5	1.6
87-88	5,851	20	338.1	191.0	1.4
88-89	4,717	16	341.2	205.1	1.4
89-90	3,737	13	344.0	220.6	1.4
90-91	2,902	10	347.0	237.1	1.3
91-92	2,206	8	358.6	254.2	1.3
92-93	1,639	6	373.0	271.3	1.2
93-94	1,190	5	386.0	288.2	1.2
94-95	843	3	399.0	305.2	1.1
95-96	584	2	412.5	322.4	1.0
96-97	394	2	425.5	340.1	1.0
97-98	259	1	438.0	358.4	0.8
98-99	166	1	451.5	377.1	0.6
99-100	103	...	464.5	396.1	...
100-101	62	...	...	415.7	...
101-102	36	...	...	436.3	...
102-103	20	...	...	458.6	...
103-104	11	...	...	482.7	...
104-105	6	...	...	508.1	...
105-106	3	...	...	534.9	...
106-107	1	...	...	564.1	...
107-108	...	...	...	595.2	...

TABLE 5. EXPECTATION OF MENTAL DISEASE AMONG NATIVE MALES IN NEW YORK STATE, 1920

Age interval, years	Of 100,000 persons born alive		Rate of mental disease per 100,000	Rate of mortality per 1,000	Expectation of mental disease
Period of life-time between two exact ages	Number alive and sane at beginning of age interval	Number becoming mentally ill in age interval	Number becoming mentally ill during age interval among 100,000 alive and sane at beginning of age interval	Number dying in age interval per 1,000 alive at beginning of interval and remaining sane during interval	Number becoming mentally ill during remainder of life of 100 alive and sane at beginning of age interval
x to $x+1$	l_x	i_x	$100{,}000\, s_x$	$1{,}000\, q_x$	$t_x = \frac{100 \Sigma_x i_x}{l_x}$
0-1	100,000	...	...	86.1	4.3
1-2	91,390	...	...	17.7	4.7
2-3	89,772	...	...	8.5	4.8
3-4	89,009	...	...	5.8	4.8
4-5	88,493	...	...	4.5	4.9
5-6	88,095	...	...	3.9	4.9
6-7	87,751	...	...	3.4	4.9
7-8	87,453	...	...	3.0	4.9
8-9	87,191	...	...	2.5	4.9
9-10	86,973	...	...	2.6	4.9
10-11	86,747	...	...	2.4	5.0
11-12	86,539	...	...	2.3	5.0
12-13	86,340	...	...	2.3	5.0
13-14	86,141	5	6.2	2.4	5.0
14-15	85,929	13	15.3	2.6	5.0
15-16	85,693	25	29.2	2.8	5.0
16-17	85,428	34	39.9	3.5	5.0
17-18	85,095	42	49.9	3.8	5.0
18-19	84,730	49	57.3	4.1	4.9
19-20	84,334	54	63.6	4.3	4.9
20-21	83,918	57	68.4	4.3	4.9
21-22	83,500	60	71.7	4.5	4.8
22-23	83,065	64	76.6	4.7	4.8
23-24	82,611	66	79.7	4.9	4.7
24-25	82,141	68	82.4	5.1	4.7
25-26	81,654	68	83.4	5.3	4.6
26-27	81,154	68	84.4	5.5	4.6
27-28	80,640	69	85.7	5.7	4.5
28-29	80,112	70	87.4	5.9	4.4
29-30	79,570	71	89.3	6.1	4.4
30-31	79,014	72	91.4	6.3	4.3
31-32	78,445	74	93.7	6.5	4.3
32-33	77,862	75	96.1	6.7	4.2
33-34	77,266	75	96.9	6.9	4.1
34-35	76,658	75	97.8	7.1	4.1
35-36	76,039	75	98.1	7.3	4.0

TABLE 5. EXPECTATION OF MENTAL DISEASE AMONG NATIVE MALES IN NEW YORK STATE, 1920—(*Continued*)

Age interval, years	Of 100,000 persons born alive		Rate of mental disease per 100,000	Rate of mortality per 1,000	Expectation of mental disease
Period of lifetime between two exact ages	Number alive and sane at beginning of age interval	Number becoming mentally ill in age interval	Number becoming mentally ill during age interval among 100,000 alive and sane at beginning of age interval	Number dying in age interval per 1,000 alive at beginning of interval and remaining sane during interval	Number becoming mentally ill during remainder of life of 100 alive and sane at beginning of age interval
x to $x+1$	l_x	i_x	$100{,}000\, s_x$	$1{,}000\, q_x$	$t_x = \frac{\sum^{100}_x i_x}{l_x}$
36-37	75,409	74	98.3	7.5	3.9
37-38	74,770	74	98.5	7.8	3.9
38-39	74,113	73	99.0	8.0	3.8
39-40	73,448	73	99.4	8.3	3.7
40-41	72,766	74	102.1	8.6	3.7
41-42	72,067	74	102.1	8.9	3.6
42-43	71,352	73	102.1	9.3	3.5
43-44	70,616	72	101.6	9.7	3.4
44-45	69,860	70	100.6	10.1	3.4
45-46	69,085	67	96.7	10.6	3.4
46-47	68,286	65	95.5	11.1	3.3
47-48	67,464	64	94.7	11.6	3.2
48-49	66,618	63	94.3	12.3	3.2
49-50	65,736	62	94.0	12.9	3.1
50-51	64,827	61	94.0	13.7	3.1
51-52	63,879	60	94.1	14.5	3.0
52-53	62,894	61	97.7	15.5	3.0
53-54	61,859	61	98.5	16.5	2.9
54-55	60,778	61	99.8	17.6	2.9
55-56	59,648	60	101.2	18.8	2.8
56-57	58,468	63	106.9	20.2	2.8
57-58	57,225	62	108.5	21.6	2.7
58-59	55,928	61	109.8	23.2	2.7
59-60	54,571	61	111.0	25.0	2.6
60-61	53,147	62	117.1	26.9	2.6
61-62	51,657	61	118.7	29.1	2.6
62-63	50,095	60	120.5	31.4	2.5
63-64	48,464	62	128.8	33.9	2.4
64-65	46,761	65	138.5	36.6	2.4
65-66	44,987	64	142.7	39.5	2.4
66-67	43,149	67	154.5	42.8	2.3
67-68	41,238	66	159.3	46.3	2.3
68-69	39,266	68	173.0	50.0	2.2
69-70	37,238	66	178.4	54.1	2.2
70-71	35,161	65	183.9	58.6	2.1
71-72	33,039	63	189.6	63.3	2.1

TABLE 5. EXPECTATION OF MENTAL DISEASE AMONG NATIVE MALES IN NEW YORK STATE, 1920—(*Continued*)

Age interval, years	Of 100,000 persons born alive		Rate of mental disease per 100,000	Rate of mortality per 1,000	Expectation of mental disease
Period of life-time between two exact ages	Number alive and sane at beginning of age interval	Number becoming mentally ill in age interval	Number becoming mentally ill during age interval among 100,000 alive and sane at beginning of age interval	Number dying in age interval per 1,000 alive at beginning of interval and remaining sane during interval	Number becoming mentally ill during remainder of life of 100 alive and sane at beginning of age interval
x to $x+1$	l_x	i_x	$100{,}000\, s_x$	$1{,}000\, q_x$	$\frac{t_x = \sum^{100}_x i_x}{l_x}$
72-73	30,889	60	195.6	68.5	2.0
73-74	28,717	58	201.9	74.1	1.9
74-75	26,535	55	208.4	80.1	1.9
75-76	24,359	52	215.0	86.5	1.8
76-77	22,204	49	221.7	93.5	1.8
77-78	20,084	46	228.3	100.9	1.7
78-79	18,016	42	234.7	109.0	1.6
79-80	16,015	39	240.5	117.6	1.6
80-81	14,097	35	245.1	126.8	1.5
81-82	12,279	31	250.6	136.7	1.4
82-83	10,574	27	257.0	147.3	1.4
83-84	8,993	24	263.0	158.6	1.4
84-85	7,547	20	269.0	170.8	1.3
85-86	6,241	17	275.0	183.7	1.2
86-87	5,081	14	281.5	197.6	1.2
87-88	4,066	12	287.6	212.4	1.2
88-89	3,193	9	293.8	228.2	1.1
89-90	2,457	7	300.0	245.0	1.1
90-91	1,850	6	306.1	262.9	1.0
91-92	1,359	4	312.5	282.0	1.0
92-93	973	3	318.5	302.4	0.9
93-94	677	2	325.0	324.0	0.9
94-95	456	2	332.0	347.0	0.9
95-96	296	1	337.0	371.5	0.7
96-97	185	1	343.6	397.5	0.5
97-98	111	...	349.8	425.1	...
98-99	64	...	356.0	454.4	...
99-100	35	...	...	485.5	...
100-101	18	...	...	518.5	...
101-102	9	...	...	553.5	...
102-103	4	...	...	590.6	...
103-104	2	...	...	629.8	...
104-105	1	...	...	671.4	...
105-106	...	...	...	...	...

TABLE 6. EXPECTATION OF MENTAL DISEASE AMONG NATIVE FEMALES IN NEW YORK STATE, 1920

Age interval, years	Of 100,000 persons born alive		Rate of mental disease per 100,000	Rate of mortality per 1,000	Expectation of mental disease
Period of lifetime between two exact ages	Number alive and sane at beginning of age interval	Number becoming mentally ill in age interval	Number becoming mentally ill during age interval among 100,000 alive and sane at beginning of age interval	Number dying in age interval per 1,000 alive at beginning of interval and remaining sane during interval	Number becoming mentally ill during remainder of life of 100 alive and sane at beginning of age interval
x to $x + 1$	l_x	i_x	$100{,}000\, s_x$	$1{,}000\, q_x$	$t_x = \frac{\sum_x^{100} i_x}{l_x}$
0-1	100,000	...	...	68.9	4.0
1-2	93,110	...	...	16.0	4.3
2-3	91,620	...	...	7.8	4.3
3-4	90,905	...	...	5.6	4.4
4-5	90,396	...	...	4.0	4.4
5-6	90,034	...	...	3.6	4.4
6-7	89,710	...	...	3.1	4.4
7-8	89,342	...	...	2.6	4.4
8-9	89,199	...	...	2.1	4.4
9-10	89,012	...	...	1.9	4.4
10-11	88,843	...	...	1.8	4.4
11-12	88,683	...	...	1.8	4.4
12-13	88,523	...	...	1.9	4.5
13-14	88,355	2	2.5	2.0	4.5
14-15	88,176	10	11.4	2.3	4.5
15-16	87,963	16	18.2	2.7	4.5
16-17	87,710	21	23.9	3.1	4.5
17-18	87,417	26	29.9	3.5	4.4
18-19	87,085	30	34.8	3.9	4.4
19-20	86,715	33	38.4	4.4	4.4
20-21	86,301	36	42.2	4.4	4.4
21-22	85,885	40	46.1	4.6	4.4
22-23	85,450	43	50.0	4.7	4.4
23-24	85,006	46	54.0	4.9	4.4
24-25	84,544	49	57.9	5.1	4.4
25-26	84,064	52	61.9	5.2	4.3
26-27	83,575	55	66.0	5.3	4.3
27-28	83,077	57	68.8	5.5	4.2
28-29	82,563	59	71.9	5.6	4.2
29-30	82,042	62	75.2	5.8	4.2
30-31	81,505	63	76.9	5.9	4.1
31-32	80,961	65	80.7	6.0	4.1
32-33	80,411	67	82.8	6.2	4.0
33-34	79,846	67	83.4	6.3	3.9
34-35	79,276	67	84.2	6.4	3.9
35-36	78,702	67	85.1	6.6	3.8

TABLE 6. EXPECTATION OF MENTAL DISEASE AMONG NATIVE FEMALES IN NEW YORK STATE, 1920—(*Continued*)

Age interval, years	Of 100,000 persons born alive		Rate of mental disease per 100,000	Rate of mortality per 1,000	Expectation of mental disease
Period of lifetime between two exact ages	Number alive and sane at beginning of age interval	Number becoming mentally ill in age interval	Number becoming mentally ill during age interval among 100,000 alive and sane at beginning of age interval	Number dying in age interval per 1,000 alive at beginning of interval and remaining sane during interval	Number becoming mentally ill during remainder of life of 100 alive and sane at beginning of age interval
x to $x+1$	l_x	i_x	$100{,}000\, s_x$	$1{,}000\, q_x$	$t_x = \dfrac{100 \sum_x i_x}{l_x}$
36-37	78,116	67	86.0	6.7	3.8
37-38	77,526	67	86.7	6.9	3.7
38-39	76,925	67	87.2	7.1	3.7
39-40	76,312	69	89.9	7.3	3.6
40-41	75,686	70	92.5	7.5	3.5
41-42	75,049	70	92.7	7.8	3.5
42-43	74,394	69	93.1	8.0	3.4
43-44	73,730	69	93.5	8.3	3.3
44-45	73,000	69	93.9	8.7	3.3
45-46	72,297	68	94.3	9.0	3.2
46-47	71,579	68	94.7	9.5	3.2
47-48	70,832	67	95.1	9.9	3.1
48-49	70,064	67	95.5	10.4	3.0
49-50	69,269	66	95.6	11.0	3.0
50-51	68,442	65	95.7	11.7	2.9
51-52	67,577	65	95.9	12.4	2.9
52-53	66,675	64	96.2	13.2	2.8
53-54	65,732	64	96.7	14.1	2.7
54-55	64,742	63	97.3	15.1	2.7
55-56	63,702	63	98.2	16.2	2.6
56-57	62,608	62	99.0	17.4	2.6
57-58	61,458	61	99.7	18.7	2.5
58-59	60,249	60	100.3	20.1	2.4
59-60	58,979	59	100.7	21.7	2.4
60-61	57,641	58	101.2	23.5	2.4
61-62	56,230	60	106.7	25.4	2.3
62-63	54,743	59	107.7	27.5	2.3
63-64	53,180	58	108.9	29.8	2.2
64-65	51,539	57	110.5	32.4	2.2
65-66	49,814	56	112.3	35.1	2.2
66-67	48,011	55	114.0	38.1	2.1
67-68	46,129	57	123.0	41.3	2.1
68-69	44,169	55	124.5	44.8	2.1
69-70	42,138	53	125.6	48.7	2.0
70-71	40,035	54	136.0	52.8	2.0
71-72	37,870	52	137.0	57.3	2.0

TABLE 6. EXPECTATION OF MENTAL DISEASE AMONG NATIVE FEMALES IN NEW YORK STATE, 1920—(*Continued*)

Age interval, years	Of 100,000 persons born alive		Rate of mental disease per 100,000	Rate of mortality per 1,000	Expectation of mental disease
Period of life-time between two exact ages	Number alive and sane at beginning of age interval	Number becoming mentally ill in age interval	Number becoming mentally ill during age interval among 100,000 alive and sane at beginning of age interval	Number dying in age interval per 1,000 alive at beginning of interval and remaining sane during interval	Number becoming mentally ill during remainder of life of 100 alive and sane at beginning of age interval
x to $x+1$	l_x	i_x	$100{,}000\, s_x$	$1{,}000\, q_x$	$t_x = \dfrac{\sum_x^{100} i_x}{l_x}$
72-73	35,651	53	149.0	62.1	1.9
73-74	33,387	50	150.2	67.4	1.9
74-75	31,090	51	164.3	73.0	1.9
75-76	28,773	52	180.2	79.1	1.9
76-77	26,449	53	198.5	85.6	1.8
77-78	24,137	49	201.7	92.7	1.8
78-79	21,855	49	225.0	100.3	1.8
79-80	19,619	45	229.8	108.4	1.7
80-81	17,452	41	234.2	117.2	1.7
81-82	15,370	37	237.8	126.5	1.6
82-83	13,393	37	274.2	136.6	1.6
83-84	11,532	32	280.1	147.3	1.5
84-85	9,806	28	284.4	158.9	1.4
85-86	8,224	23	285.5	171.2	1.4
86-87	6,797	20	296.5	184.4	1.4
87-88	5,527	17	307.8	198.4	1.4
88-89	4,417	14	319.0	213.4	1.3
89-90	3,463	11	330.2	229.5	1.3
90-91	2,660	9	343.0	246.5	1.2
91-92	1,998	7	356.5	264.7	1.2
92-93	1,464	5	369.5	284.1	1.2
93-94	1,044	4	382.0	304.8	1.1
94-95	723	3	394.5	326.7	1.1
95-96	485	2	427.0	350.1	1.0
96-97	314	1	456.0	374.9	1.0
97-98	196	1	485.0	401.3	1.0
98-99	117	1	520.0	429.3	0.9
99-100	66	...	549.0	459.0	...
100-101	36	...	...	490.5	...
101-102	18	...	...	524.0	...
102-103	9	...	...	559.4	...
103-104	4	...	...	597.0	...
104-105	2	...	...	636.8	...
105-106	1	...	...	678.9	...

TABLE 7. EXPECTATION OF MENTAL DISEASE AMONG FOREIGN-BORN MALES IN NEW YORK STATE, 1920

Age interval, years	Of 100,000 persons born alive		Rate of mental disease per 100,000	Rate of mortality per 1,000	Expectation of mental disease
Period of lifetime between two exact ages	Number alive and sane at beginning of age interval	Number becoming mentally ill in age interval	Number becoming mentally ill during age interval among 100,000 alive and sane at beginning of age interval	Number dying in age interval per 1,000 alive at beginning of interval and remaining sane during interval	Number becoming mentally ill during remainder of life of 100 alive and sane at beginning of age interval
x to $x+1$	l_x	i_x	$100{,}000\,s_x$	$1{,}000\,q_x$	$t_x = \frac{\sum^{100}_{x} i_x}{l_x}$
0-1	100,000	...	...	84.3	5.4
1-2	91,570	...	...	17.6	5.8
2-3	89,958	...	...	8.5	6.0
3-4	89,193	...	...	5.9	6.0
4-5	88,667	...	...	4.6	6.0
5-6	88,259	...	...	4.8	6.1
6-7	87,835	...	...	3.9	6.1
7-8	87,492	...	...	3.4	6.1
8-9	87,195	...	...	2.8	6.1
9-10	86,951	...	...	2.4	6.2
10-11	86,742	...	...	2.2	6.2
11-12	86,551	...	...	2.1	6.2
12-13	86,369	...	...	2.2	6.2
13-14	86,179	...	...	2.5	6.2
14-15	85,964	52	60.2	2.8	6.2
15-16	85,671	74	86.1	3.3	6.2
16-17	85,315	90	106.0	3.8	6.1
17-18	84,901	102	120.6	4.3	6.1
18-19	84,434	105	123.9	4.7	6.0
19-20	83,933	112	132.9	4.8	5.9
20-21	83,409	110	131.8	5.3	5.8
21-22	82,858	108	130.9	5.3	5.7
22-23	82,311	107	130.5	5.4	5.6
23-24	81,760	107	130.3	5.4	5.5
24-25	81,212	106	130.0	5.5	5.4
25-26	80,660	104	129.2	5.6	5.3
26-27	80,105	101	126.4	5.7	5.2
27-28	79,548	98	123.4	5.8	5.1
28-29	78,989	97	123.0	5.9	5.0
29-30	78,426	97	124.0	6.0	4.9
30-31	77,859	96	123.4	6.1	4.9
31-32	77,289	96	123.8	6.2	4.8
32-33	76,714	96	124.9	6.4	4.7
33-34	76,128	95	124.4	6.5	4.6
34-35	75,539	93	122.6	6.7	4.5
35-36	74,941	93	124.0	7.0	4.4

TABLE 7. EXPECTATION OF MENTAL DISEASE AMONG FOREIGN-BORN MALES IN NEW YORK STATE, 1920—(*Continued*)

Age interval, years	Of 100,000 persons born alive		Rate of mental disease per 100,000	Rate of mortality per 1,000	Expectation of mental disease
Period of lifetime between two exact ages	Number alive and sane at beginning of age interval	Number becoming mentally ill in age interval	Number becoming mentally ill during age interval among 100,000 alive and sane at beginning of age interval	Number dying in age interval per 1,000 alive at beginning of interval and remaining sane during interval	Number becoming mentally ill during remainder of life of 100 alive and sane at beginning of age interval
x to $x+1$	l_x	i_x	$100,000\, s_x$	$1,000\, q_x$	$t_x = \frac{100 \sum_x i_x}{l_x}$
36-37	74,324	91	123.1	7.2	4.3
37-38	73,699	90	122.0	7.5	4.2
38-39	73,057	90	123.3	7.8	4.2
39-40	72,398	88	121.9	8.1	4.1
40-41	71,724	89	123.4	8.5	4.0
41-42	71,026	85	119.8	8.9	3.9
42-43	70,310	84	119.5	9.3	3.8
43-44	69,573	82	117.3	9.8	3.7
44-45	68,810	80	115.6	10.4	3.7
45-46	68,015	78	114.2	11.0	3.6
46-47	67,190	74	109.4	11.7	3.5
47-48	66,331	73	110.7	12.5	3.4
48-49	65,430	71	108.0	13.3	3.4
49-50	64,490	70	108.5	14.2	3.3
50-51	63,505	69	108.9	15.2	3.3
51-52	62,472	68	109.5	16.3	3.2
52-53	61,387	68	110.5	17.4	3.1
53-54	60,252	67	112.0	18.7	3.1
54-55	59,060	67	113.7	20.1	3.0
55-56	57,807	67	116.0	21.6	3.3
56-57	56,493	67	118.4	23.3	2.9
57-58	55,111	66	120.4	25.1	2.9
58-59	53,663	69	128.3	27.0	2.9
59-60	52,147	68	130.1	29.1	2.8
60-61	50,564	67	131.8	31.4	2.8
61-62	48,911	65	133.4	33.8	2.7
62-63	47,195	67	143.0	36.5	2.7
63-64	45,408	66	145.4	39.3	2.6
64-65	43,560	68	157.1	42.4	2.6
65-66	41,648	67	160.3	45.7	2.5
66-67	39,681	69	174.4	49.2	2.5
67-68	37,663	67	178.2	53.0	2.4
68-69	35,603	69	194.8	57.1	2.4
69-70	33,505	67	199.3	61.5	2.4
70-71	31,382	64	203.4	66.2	2.3
71-72	29,245	61	207.0	71.2	2.2

TABLE 7. EXPECTATION OF MENTAL DISEASE AMONG FOREIGN-BORN MALES IN NEW YORK STATE, 1920—(*Continued*)

Age interval, years	Of 100,000 persons born alive		Rate of mental disease per 100,000	Rate of mortality per 1,000	Expectation of mental disease
Period of lifetime between two exact ages	Number alive and sane at beginning of age interval	Number becoming mentally ill in age interval	Number becoming mentally ill during age interval among 100,000 alive and sane at beginning of age interval	Number dying in age interval per 1,000 alive at beginning of interval and remaining sane during interval	Number becoming mentally ill during remainder of life of 100 alive and sane at beginning of age interval
x to $x+1$	l_x	i_x	$100{,}000\, s_x$	$1{,}000\, q_x$	$\dfrac{t_x = \sum_x^{100} i_x}{l_x}$
72-73	27,106	57	209.6	76.6	2.2
73-74	24,977	53	210.4	82.4	2.2
74-75	22,870	53	232.1	88.5	2.1
75-76	20,798	50	239.0	95.1	2.1
76-77	18,775	46	247.0	102.1	2.0
77-78	16,817	43	254.3	109.5	2.0
78-79	14,937	40	271.0	117.5	2.0
79-80	13,147	38	287.5	126.0	1.9
80-81	11,457	33	291.0	135.0	1.9
81-82	9,882	30	306.0	144.7	1.9
82-83	8,426	28	327.1	154.9	1.8
83-84	7,097	24	334.0	165.8	1.8
84-85	5,900	21	360.5	177.3	1.7
85-86	4,837	18	370.5	189.6	1.7
86-87	3,905	15	378.0	202.7	1.6
87-88	3,101	12	386.0	216.5	1.5
88-89	2,420	9	390.5	231.2	1.4
89-90	1,854	7	392.5	246.7	1.4
90-91	1,391	6	433.0	263.2	1.4
91-92	1,020	5	449.4	280.7	1.4
92-93	730	3	464.0	299.2	1.2
93-94	509	2	479.0	318.8	1.2
94-95	345	2	493.0	339.5	1.2
95-96	227	1	511.0	361.4	0.9
96-97	144	1	629.0	384.6	0.7
97-98	88	...	547.0	409.1	...
98-99	52	...	564.0	435.0	...
99-100	29	...	572.0	462.4	...
100-101	16	...	...	491.2	...
101-102	8	...	...	521.7	...
102-103	4	...	...	553.9	...
103-104	2	...	...	587.8	...
104-105	1	...	...	623.6	...
105-106	...	...	...	...	...

TABLE 8. EXPECTATION OF MENTAL DISEASE AMONG FOREIGN-BORN FEMALES IN NEW YORK STATE, 1920

Age interval, years	Of 100,000 persons born alive		Rate of Mental disease per 100,000	Rate of mortality per 1,000	Expectation of mental disease
Period of life-time between two exact ages	Number alive and sane at beginning of age interval	Number becoming mentally ill in age interval	Number becoming mentally ill during age interval among 100,000 alive and sane at beginning of age interval	Number dying in age interval per 1,000 alive at beginning of interval and remaining sane during interval	Number becoming mentally ill during remainder of life of 100 alive and sane at beginning of age interval
x to $x+1$	l_x	i_x	$100{,}000\, s_x$	$1{,}000\, q_x$	$t_x = \frac{100 \sum_x i_x}{l_x}$
0-1	100,000	...	...	67.3	5.2
1-2	93,270	...	...	15.8	5.6
2-3	91,796	...	...	7.7	5.7
3-4	91,089	...	...	5.6	5.7
4-5	90,579	...	...	4.1	5.7
5-6	90,208	...	...	3.6	5.8
6-7	89,883	...	...	3.1	5.8
7-8	89,604	...	...	2.6	5.8
8-9	89,371	...	...	2.2	5.8
9-10	89,174	...	...	1.9	5.8
10-11	89,005	...	...	1.8	5.8
11-12	88,845	...	...	1.8	5.9
12-13	88,685	...	...	1.9	5.9
13-14	88,516	...	...	2.1	5.9
14-15	88,330	44	50.0	2.3	5.9
15-16	88,083	46	51.7	2.7	5.9
16-17	87,799	52	59.0	3.1	5.8
17-18	87,475	54	62.0	3.5	5.8
18-19	87,115	57	65.2	3.8	5.7
19-20	86,727	57	65.7	4.3	5.7
20-21	86,297	62	71.3	4.7	5.7
21-22	85,830	65	76.0	4.9	5.6
22-23	85,345	68	79.6	5.0	5.6
23-24	84,851	73	85.7	5.0	5.5
24-25	84,354	76	89.9	5.0	5.4
25-26	83,857	79	94.1	5.0	5.4
26-27	83,359	84	101.2	5.1	5.4
27-28	82,850	85	102.7	5.1	5.3
28-29	82,343	87	105.3	5.1	5.2
29-30	81,836	87	105.7	5.2	5.1
30-31	81,324	87	106.8	5.3	5.1
31-32	80,806	86	106.8	5.4	5.0
32-33	80,284	86	106.8	5.5	4.9
33-34	79,757	85	107.0	5.6	4.8
34-35	79,226	85	107.0	5.8	4.8
35-36	78,682	85	107.5	5.9	4.7

TABLE 8. EXPECTATION OF MENTAL DISEASE AMONG FOREIGN-BORN FEMALES IN NEW YORK STATE, 1920—(*Continued*)

Age interval, years	Of 100,000 persons born alive		Rate of mental disease per 100,000	Rate of mortality per 1,000	Expectation of mental disease
Period of life-time between two exact ages	Number alive and sane at beginning of age interval	Number becoming mentally ill in age interval	Number becoming mentally ill during age interval among 100,000 alive and sane at beginning of age interval	Number dying in age interval per 1,000 alive at beginning of interval and remaining sane during interval	Number becoming mentally ill during remainder of life of 100 alive and sane at beginning of age interval
x to $x+1$	l_x	i_x	$100{,}000\, s_x$	$1{,}000\, q_x$	$t_x = \frac{\overset{100}{\Sigma}\, i_x}{l_x}$
36-37	78,133	84	107.5	6.1	4.6
37-38	77,573	83	107.6	6.3	4.5
38-39	77,002	83	108.0	6.6	4.4
39-40	76,411	83	108.0	6.9	4.4
40-41	75,801	82	108.5	7.2	4.3
41-42	75,174	82	108.5	7.6	4.3
42-43	74,521	81	109.0	8.0	4.2
43-44	73,844	80	109.0	8.5	4.1
44-45	73,137	80	109.5	9.0	4.0
45-46	72,399	85	117.1	9.6	4.0
46-47	71,620	84	117.6	10.2	3.9
47-48	70,806	83	117.8	10.9	3.8
48-49	69,952	85	122.0	11.7	3.7
49-50	69,050	84	122.0	12.6	3.7
50-51	68,096	83	122.0	13.5	3.6
51-52	67,095	82	122.0	14.2	3.5
52-53	66,061	81	122.3	15.7	3.4
53-54	64,944	80	123.1	16.9	3.4
54-55	63,768	76	118.9	18.3	3.3
55-56	62,526	75	119.9	19.8	3.3
56-57	61,214	74	120.9	21.4	3.2
57-58	59,832	72	121.0	23.1	3.2
58-59	58,380	71	121.6	25.0	3.1
59-60	56,851	69	122.0	27.1	3.1
60-61	55,243	69	124.8	29.3	3.1
61-62	53,557	68	127.7	31.7	3.0
62-63	51,793	70	135.4	34.3	3.0
63-64	49,949	72	143.7	37.1	3.0
64-65	48,027	73	152.8	40.1	2.9
65-66	46,031	75	162.7	43.4	2.9
66-67	43,962	76	173.6	46.9	2.9
67-68	41,828	78	185.7	50.6	2.8
68-69	39,637	78	198.0	54.7	2.8
69-70	37,395	80	214.4	59.0	2.8
70-71	35,113	76	217.0	63.6	2.7
71-72	32,809	77	234.9	68.6	2.7

TABLE 8. EXPECTATION OF MENTAL DISEASE AMONG FOREIGN-BORN FEMALES IN NEW YORK STATE, 1920—(*Continued*)

Age interval, years	Of 100,000 persons born alive		Rate of mental disease per 100,000	Rate of mortality per 1,000	Expectation of mental disease
Period of life-time between two exact ages	Number alive and sane at beginning of age interval	Number becoming mentally ill in age interval	Number becoming mentally ill during age interval among 100,000 alive and sane at beginning of age interval	Number dying in age interval per 1,000 alive at beginning of interval and remaining sane during interval	Number becoming mentally ill during remainder of life of 100 alive and sane at beginning of age interval
x to $x + 1$	l_x	i_x	$100{,}000\, s_x$	$1{,}000\, q_x$	$t_x = \frac{\sum^{100} i_x}{l_x}$
72-73	30,487	73	238.3	73.9	2.6
73-74	28,166	73	259.9	79.6	2.6
74-75	25,857	68	264.5	85.7	2.5
75-76	23,579	63	268.9	92.1	2.4
76-77	21,350	64	297.5	99.1	2.4
77-78	19,177	58	303.4	106.5	2.4
78-79	17,083	53	308.4	114.4	2.3
79-80	15,082	52	346.7	122.8	2.3
80-81	13,184	47	353.4	131.7	2.2
81-82	11,407	41	358.9	141.2	2.2
82-83	9,761	37	377.0	151.3	2.1
83-84	8,253	32	390.0	162.1	2.1
84-85	6,888	28	404.0	173.5	2.0
85-86	5,670	23	414.0	185.6	1.9
86-87	4,599	20	425.5	198.5	1.9
87-88	3,670	16	438.0	212.2	1.8
88-89	2,879	13	450.0	226.7	1.8
89-90	2,216	10	465.0	242.0	1.7
90-91	1,672	8	482.0	258.3	1.7
91-92	1,234	6	500.0	275.6	1.6
92-93	890	5	523.0	293.8	1.6
93-94	625	3	547.0	313.2	1.4
94-95	427	2	572.0	333.6	1.4
95-96	283	2	598.0	355.2	1.4
96-97	181	1	624.0	378.1	1.1
97-98	112	1	648.0	402.2	0.9
98-99	66	...	680.0	427.7	0.6
99-100	38	...	710.0	454.7	...
100-101	21	...	...	454.7	...
101-102	11	...	...	513.2	...
102-103	5	...	...	544.8	...
103-104	2	...	...	578.3	...
104-105	1	...	...	613.5	...
105-106	...	...	...	...	...

CHAPTER III

Outcome of Mental Diseases in the United States*

The special census of hospitals for mental disease taken by the Federal Census Bureau as of January 1, 1923, gave more comprehensive data concerning the outcome of the various forms of mental disease in the country as a whole than had hitherto been available. The census covered the patients resident in institutions for mental disease on the date of the enumeration and the first admissions, readmissions, discharges, and deaths of the calendar year 1922.

In taking the census, individual schedules were filled out by persons officially connected with the institutions who were engaged for this purpose by the Census Bureau. Returns were thus secured from 526 institutions for mental disease, of which 163 were state hospitals, 2 government hospitals, 148 other public hospitals, and 213 private institutions. Montana was the only state that failed to submit data concerning individual patients in time for tabulation; the general movement of patients, however, was reported by all states.

Movement of Patient Population

The great significance of these institutions is indicated by the magnitude of their yearly operations. The patients on books January 1, 1922, embraced 258,421 resident patients and 21,137 paroles. The incoming patients during the year comprised 73,063 first admissions and 16,392 readmissions; the departures included 52,777 discharges and 25,656 deaths. On January 1, 1923, the resident patients numbered 267,617 and the paroles, 22,839. The net increase in resident patients during the year was 9,196[1] and in paroles 1,701.

From the above data we find that for each 1,000 patients resident in hospitals at the beginning of the year, there were during the year 283 first admissions, 63 readmissions, 204 discharges, and 99 deaths. The increase in resident patients per 1,000 was 36 and in paroles 7.

*Originally published in *Mental Hygiene*, October, 1925.

(1) In the returns, the outgoing transfers exceeded the incoming transfers by 124. These were probably sent to other types of institutions.

TABLE 1. MOVEMENT OF PATIENTS IN HOSPITALS FOR MENTAL DISEASE IN UNITED STATES, BY PSYCHOSIS AND SEX, 1922*

Psychoses	First admissions			Readmissions			Discharges			Deaths			Resident patients, January 1, 1923		
	M.	F.	T.	M.	F.	T.	M.	F.	T.	M.	F.	T.	M.	F.	T.
Traumatic	197	32	229	27	4	31	137	28	165	33	9	42	469	52	521
Senile	3,563	3,282	6,845	210	265	475	828	911	1,739	2,643	2,431	5,074	5,946	7,639	13,585
With cerebral arteriosclerosis	2,233	1,205	3,438	170	108	278	559	354	913	1,530	820	2,350	2,706	1,713	4,419
General paralysis	5,076	1,218	6,294	505	138	643	1,421	380	1,801	3,816	869	4,685	7,318	2,076	9,394
With cerebral syphilis	637	256	893	87	35	122	297	121	418	278	101	379	1,190	620	1,810
With Huntington's chorea	45	52	97	12	4	16	16	18	34	35	35	70	146	171	317
With brain tumor	35	26	61	3	2	5	25	13	38	19	14	33	25	24	49
With other brain or nervous diseases	387	256	643	49	22	71	198	111	309	169	117	286	620	440	1,060
Alcoholic	2,427	266	2,693	536	62	598	2,314	236	2,550	331	82	413	6,252	1,144	7,396
Due to drugs and other exogenous toxins	372	243	615	98	60	158	436	255	691	34	33	67	313	241	554
With pellagra	125	295	420	16	26	42	83	146	229	76	158	234	141	366	507
With other somatic diseases	738	1,068	1,806	63	98	161	396	666	1,062	326	366	692	778	1,200	1,978
Manic-depressive	4,880	6,513	11,393	1,884	2,672	4,556	5,236	6,766	12,002	1,164	1,481	2,645	17,129	23,622	40,751
Involution melancholia	560	1,243	1,803	90	237	327	401	963	1,364	239	381	620	1,807	3,956	5,763
Dementia præcox	8,950	6,576	15,526	2,479	1,922	4,401	6,785	4,659	11,444	1,930	2,018	3,948	60,653	53,587	114,240
Paranoia or paranoid conditions	873	1,008	1,881	171	260	431	681	749	1,430	175	227	402	5,683	6,270	11,953
Epileptic psychoses	1,121	692	1,813	247	140	387	647	364	1,011	606	413	1,019	5,061	4,094	9,155
Psychoneuroses and neuroses	1,658	1,119	2,777	615	243	858	2,258	1,196	3,454	33	52	85	1,220	1,131	2,351
With psychopathic personality	585	329	914	184	127	311	602	288	890	49	29	78	1,675	1,208	2,883
With mental deficiency	1,076	823	1,899	238	166	404	731	437	1,168	213	201	414	6,378	5,564	11,942
Undiagnosed psychoses	2,363	1,831	4,194	291	260	551	1,577	1,232	2,809	668	561	1,229	7,738	6,497	14,235
Without psychosis	3,616	1,541	5,157	956	308	1,264	4,058	1,505	5,563	346	223	569	5,700	3,799	9,499
Unascertained	197	88	285	18	25	43	113	107	220	56	46	102	826	641	1,467
Total	41,714	29,962	71,676	8,949	7,184	16,133	29,799	21,505	51,304	14,769	10,667	25,436	139,774	126,055	265,829

*Transfers omitted.

Individual schedules were received by the Census Bureau for 265,829 resident patients, 71,676 first admissions, 16,133 readmissions, 51,304 discharges, and 25,436 deaths.

The movement of patients by psychoses tabulated from these schedules is shown in Table 1. It will be seen that in the several psychotic groups the relation of resident patients to admissions, discharges, and deaths varies greatly. Groups of psychoses having a relatively high ratio of first admissions to resident patients are cerebral arteriosclerosis, general paralysis, brain tumor, with other brain or nervous diseases, drug and other toxic psychoses, with pellagra, and psychoneuroses and neuroses.

Readmissions are most prominent in the alcoholic, manic-depressive, and dementia præcox groups, although a considerable number is found in each of the other clinical groups.

More than half of the discharges are furnished by the manic-depressive, dementia præcox, and psychoneurosis groups.

Deaths are relatively most numerous in the organic groups, although a considerable proportion are found in the so-called functional groups. Closer comparisons of deaths in the several psychoses are made in a later table which gives classified death rates in each group.

Discharges

Of the 51,304 discharges for whom individual schedules were received, 11,935, or 23.3 per cent, were discharged as recovered; 23,683, or 46.2 per cent, as improved; 9,796, or 19.1 per cent, as unimproved; 4,943, or 9.6 per cent, as without psychosis; and 947, or 1.8 per cent, as unascertained.

In the instructions to enumerators the above terms denoting the condition of the patients on discharge were explained as follows:

"*Recovered* indicates the condition of a patient who has regained his normal health, so that he may be considered as having practically the same mental status as he had previous to the onset of his psychosis.

"*Improved* denotes any degree of mental gain less than recovered.

"*Unimproved,* as the term implies, denotes no mental gain.

"*Without psychosis* is a term applicable to persons discharged who had been admitted to a hospital without having had a psychosis."

The general recovery rate of patients per 100 admissions for the whole United States was 13.6; the rate for the males was 12.5, and for the females 15.1. The rate of discharges as improved for all patients was 27.0; for males, 26.2; and for females, 28.0. The higher recovery and improvement rates among females are due principally to the excess of males in the general paralysis group, which yielded practically no recoveries, and to the excess of females in the manic-depressive group, which yielded a high percentage of recoveries.

Table 2 sets forth the rates of discharges of the several classes as determined from the discharge schedules received from the several states. Judging from the wide variations shown in the table, it seems probable that the terms denoting condition on discharge were not uniformly applied. However, as the rates are affected both by the number of admissions and the number of discharges, considerable variation would be expected.

Some states, like Illinois, Massachusetts, and Wisconsin, seem to have adopted a conservative policy in regard to discharging patients as recovered; their recovery rates, therefore, are out of line as compared with those of most of the other states. As would be expected, many states that have low recovery rates have relatively high improvement rates.

The rates of patients discharged as unimproved are influenced by many factors. A considerable portion of the patients thus discharged are returned to their homes in foreign countries or in other states.

The group of discharges included under the heading "otherwise discharged" equals 6.7 per cent of the admissions. This group comprises the nonpsychotic cases and some psychotic cases that should have been designated as recovered, improved, or unimproved.

The general average rate of discharges per 100 of all admissions, excluding transfers, is 58.4. As the deviations from this average rate in the more populous states are not large, the rate seems to be an approximation of the normal relation between admissions and discharges of patients of all clinical groups taken together.

TABLE 2. RATES PER 100 ADMISSIONS OF PATIENTS DISCHARGED FROM HOSPITALS FOR MENTAL DISEASE DURING 1922, CLASSIFIED BY CONDITION ON DISCHARGE AND BY STATES

States	Total	Recovered	Improved	Unimproved	Otherwise discharged*
Alabama	64.8	6.5	37.0	19.8	1.5
Arizona	17.4	8.5	3.8	0.9	4.2
Arkansas	70.9	35.1	16.0	2.6	17.2
California	65.5	18.6	27.0	10.2	9.7
Colorado	53.2	13.8	28.0	9.7	1.8
Connecticut	66.2	13.2	25.4	12.7	14.9
Delaware	57.3	17.3	35.5	3.6	0.9
District of Columbia	53.7	15.0	10.6	19.4	8.7
Florida	32.1	10.5	13.5	2.0	6.2
Georgia	75.9	17.0	37.7	18.3	2.8
Idaho	50.6	7.3	36.5	5.1	1.7
Illinois	62.3	10.1	36.0	7.1	9.2
Indiana	48.8	15.1	29.2	4.1	0.5
Iowa	67.6	13.9	18.6	22.6	12.6
Kansas	55.9	7.8	36.1	8.1	3.9
Kentucky	55.1	7.2	36.0	4.9	7.0
Louisiana	57.1	15.7	20.7	12.8	8.0
Maine	55.7	16.8	17.4	11.6	9.9
Maryland	65.2	10.3	37.9	15.2	1.7
Massachusetts	65.3	5.8	23.3	26.3	9.9
Michigan	60.6	12.1	26.8	16.4	5.3
Minnesota	57.6	11.4	29.3	5.0	12.0
Mississippi	64.6	13.4	29.0	11.8	10.4
Missouri	54.0	11.0	26.4	7.7	8.8
Nebraska	52.1	3.7	25.4	8.7	14.4
Nevada	72.7	31.8	22.7	6.8	11.4
New Hampshire	57.4	10.7	26.4	9.8	10.4
New Jersey	51.3	15.1	23.9	7.1	5.2
New Mexico	48.0	...	44.8	...	3.2
New York	54.1	17.8	23.3	9.2	3.8
North Carolina	54.4	13.4	28.8	6.1	6.1
North Dakota	54.2	20.8	22.2	10.6	0.7
Ohio	56.5	16.1	25.2	10.0	5.2
Oklahoma	58.1	8.8	37.4	6.7	5.3
Oregon	45.3	20.3	17.2	7.6	0.2
Pennsylvania	53.6	12.4	29.8	8.7	2.7
Rhode Island	48.5	12.5	26.9	7.0	2.1
South Carolina	60.3	18.2	28.6	5.6	7.9
South Dakota	47.7	9.4	30.6	4.7	3.0
Tennessee	64.6	8.7	32.7	13.7	9.6
Texas	57.6	20.1	21.3	11.1	5.1
Utah	70.1	1.2	60.6	7.5	0.8
Vermont	54.0	9.5	26.5	10.0	8.1
Virginia	60.5	25.7	19.9	7.1	7.9
Washington	53.0	16.6	23.2	10.7	2.5
West Virginia	60.4	20.0	29.3	7.6	3.5
Wisconsin	58.5	8.2	28.9	14.8	6.7
Wyoming	21.9	6.0	3.0	9.5	3.5
Total	58.4	13.6	27.0	11.2	6.7

*Includes those discharged as without psychosis and unascertained cases.

Discharges in the Separate Groups of Psychoses

Table 3 gives rates of discharges, classified by psychosis, sex, and condition on discharge for the whole United States, excepting Montana. Groups of psychoses with high rates of discharges are the alcoholic, drug, manic-depressive, psychoneuroses and neuroses, and with psychopathic personality; those with low rates are the senile, arteriosclerotic, general paralysis, with Huntington's chorea, with other brain and nervous diseases, with pellagra, and epilepsy.

Recovery rates naturally vary greatly in the several groups of psychoses. The highest recovery rate is found in the drug group, the next highest in the alcoholic group, and the next in the manic-depressive group. Very few recoveries are reported in the so-called organic groups, but a large proportion of the patients in these groups improve sufficiently to be discharged. In the large dementia præcox group the recovery rate in 1922 was only 6.4 per

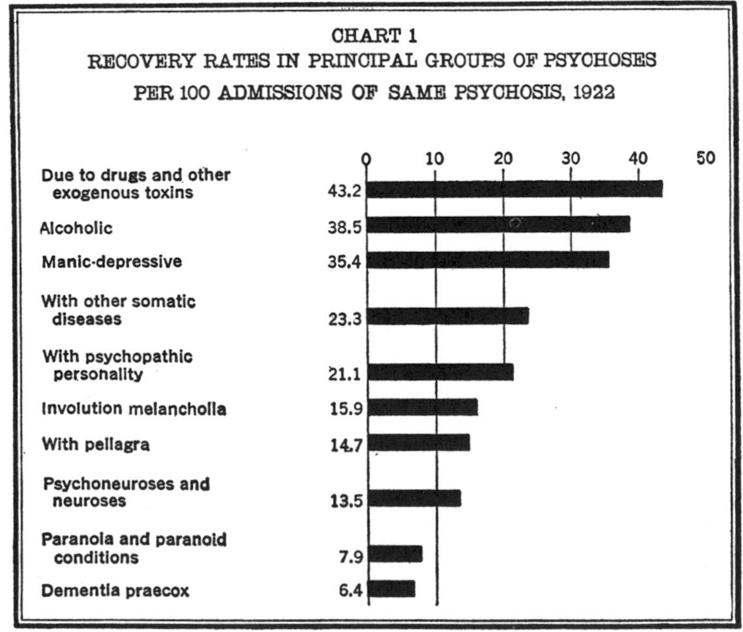

TABLE 3. RATES PER 100 ADMISSIONS WITH SAME PSYCHOSIS OF PATIENTS DISCHARGED FROM HOSPITALS FOR MENTAL DISEASE DURING 1922, CLASSIFIED BY SEX AND CONDITION ON DISCHARGE

Psychoses	Total			Recovered			Improved			Unimproved			Otherwise discharged*		
	M.	F.	T.	M.	F.	T.	M.	F.	T.	M.	F.	T.	M.	F.	T.
Traumatic	61.2	77.8	63.5	17.9	36.1	20.4	28.6	33.3	29.2	13.4	8.3	12.7	1.3	...	1.2
Senile	21.9	25.7	23.8	1.4	1.3	1.3	11.4	14.3	12.8	8.6	9.6	9.1	0.6	0.5	0.5
With cerebral arteriosclerosis	23.3	27.0	24.6	2.0	2.2	2.0	14.2	17.9	15.5	6.5	6.5	6.5	0.6	0.4	0.5
General paralysis	25.5	28.0	26.0	0.5	0.8	0.5	12.9	16.3	13.5	11.3	10.5	11.1	0.8	0.4	0.7
With cerebral syphilis	41.0	41.6	41.2	5.4	5.2	5.3	23.8	25.1	24.1	11.0	11.3	11.1	0.8	...	0.6
With Huntington's chorea	28.1	32.1	30.1	1.8	1.8	1.8	12.3	21.4	16.8	12.3	8.9	10.6	1.8	...	0.9
With brain tumor	65.8	46.4	57.6	...	3.6	1.5	21.1	17.9	19.7	44.7	25.0	36.4	...	...	...
With other brain or nervous diseases	45.4	39.9	43.8	5.7	3.2	4.8	22.0	19.4	21.0	17.2	15.8	16.7	0.5	1.4	0.8
Alcoholic	78.1	72.0	77.5	39.5	29.6	38.5	30.0	31.7	30.1	5.0	8.8	5.4	3.6	1.8	3.5
Due to drugs and other exogenous toxins	92.8	84.2	89.4	43.4	42.9	43.2	36.2	33.3	35.1	9.4	6.6	8.3	3.8	1.3	2.8
With pellagra	58.9	45.5	49.6	17.7	13.4	14.7	31.2	25.2	27.1	9.2	6.9	7.6	0.7	...	0.2
With other somatic diseases	49.4	57.1	54.0	20.7	25.1	23.3	23.0	23.2	23.1	4.9	7.6	6.5	0.9	1.2	1.1
Manic-depressive	77.4	73.7	75.3	36.7	34.4	35.4	31.5	31.4	31.4	8.2	7.2	7.6	0.9	0.6	0.8
Involution melancholia	61.7	65.1	64.0	12.8	17.3	15.9	32.8	35.3	34.6	15.8	11.4	12.8	0.3	1.0	0.8
Dementia præcox	59.4	54.8	57.4	6.3	6.6	6.4	33.8	33.3	33.6	17.6	13.7	16.0	1.6	1.2	1.4
Paranoia or paranoid conditions	65.3	59.1	61.9	10.7	5.6	7.9	31.1	33.5	32.4	22.3	19.2	20.6	1.1	0.7	0.9
Epileptic	47.2	43.8	45.9	4.7	6.1	5.2	25.7	24.0	25.1	15.4	13.1	14.5	1.4	0.5	1.0
Psychoneuroses and neuroses	99.3	87.8	95.0	9.1	20.7	13.5	68.8	49.3	61.5	16.6	13.9	15.6	4.8	3.9	4.5
With psychopathic personality	78.3	63.2	72.7	26.4	12.3	21.1	32.6	37.5	34.4	15.9	12.7	14.7	3.4	0.7	2.4
With mental deficiency	55.6	44.2	50.7	11.7	9.9	10.9	27.3	22.0	25.1	15.0	10.2	12.9	1.6	2.0	1.8
Undiagnosed psychoses	59.4	58.9	59.2	10.4	11.5	10.9	31.1	31.3	31.2	13.3	13.2	13.3	4.6	3.0	3.9
Without psychosis	88.7	81.4	86.6	4.9	7.1	5.6	5.4	6.2	5.7	3.8	3.2	3.6	74.5	64.9	71.8
Unascertained	53.0	94.7	67.4	4.7	5.3	4.9	11.6	30.1	18.0	8.4	13.3	10.1	28.4	46.0	34.5
Total	58.8	57.9	58.4	12.5	15.1	13.6	26.2	28.0	27.0	11.7	10.4	11.2	8.4	4.4	6.7

*Includes those discharged as without psychosis and unascertained cases.

100 admissions, but the discharged improved rate was 33.6 and the discharged unimproved rate 16.0.

Comparing rates of cases discharged as improved, we find the highest rate in the psychoneuroses group and the next highest in the drug group. Other groups with high rates are the involution melancholia, with psychopathic personality, and alcoholic groups.

Female patients fare somewhat better than male patients in being discharged, both the recovery and improvement rates of the former being the higher. As previously mentioned, the females gain an advantage over the males by being represented by few cases in the general paralysis group. Some of the noteworthy differences in recovery and improvement rates per 100 admissions among males and females are seen in the following comparisons:

Psychoses	Recovery rate		Improvement rate	
	Males	Females	Males	Females
Alcoholic	39.5	29.6	30.0	31.7
With other somatic diseases	20.7	25.1	23.0	23.2
Involution melancholia	12.8	17.3	32.8	35.3
Paranoia or paranoid conditions	10.7	5.6	31.1	33.5
Psychoneuroses and neuroses	9.1	20.7	68.8	49.3
With psychopathic personality	26.4	12.3	32.6	37.5

The causes of these differences in the rates in the two sexes are not fully known.

Table 4 shows the rate per 100 admissions of patients discharged as recovered classified by psychosis and age. The recovery rate for the country as a whole in the successive age groups below 70 was as follows: under 15 years, 4.8; 15 to 19 years, 13.4; 20 to 24 years, 15.2; 25 to 29 years, 14.1; 30 to 34 years, 14.4; 35 to 39 years, 16.7; 40 to 44 years, 16.8; 45 to 49 years, 15.9; 50 to 54 years, 15.6; 55 to 59 years, 13.5; 60 to 64 years, 10.7; 65 to 69 years, 6.9. It will be noted that the highest rates of recovery occur between 35 and 45 years and that the rates vary comparatively little between the ages of 15 and 60.

TABLE 4. RATE PER 100 ADMISSIONS OF SAME PSYCHOSIS AND AGE OF PATIENTS DISCHARGED AS RECOVERED FROM HOSPITALS FOR MENTAL DISEASE DURING 1922

Psychoses	Total	Under 15 years	15 to 19 years	20 to 24 years	25 to 29 years	30 to 34 years	35 to 39 years	40 to 44 years	45 to 49 years	50 to 54 years	55 to 59 years	60 to 64 years	65 to 69 years	70 to 74 years	75 to 79 years	80 years and over
Traumatic	20.4	...	10.0	21.1	24.0	16.1	20.0	32.3	19.2	40.0	12.0	15.4	7.1	...	...	...
Senile	1.3	...	...	...	...	...	...	...	6.3	6.3	2.4	2.0	1.3	1.2	1.2	0.1
With cerebral arteriosclerosis	2.0	...	...	...	25.0	33.3	...	2.1	4.9	5.3	2.8	2.2	1.5	1.1	0.9	...
General paralysis	0.5	...	...	1.1	1.2	0.4	0.3	0.5	0.6	0.8	0.4	0.7	0.7	...	...	...
With cerebral syphilis	5.3	...	20.0	15.4	5.7	3.2	7.3	7.3	5.3	2.8	2.9	...	5.7	...	...	...
With Huntington's chorea	1.8	...	...	33.3	...	...	12.5	...	...	...	...	...	...	...	...	...
With brain tumor	1.5	...	...	...	...	...	...	...	...	12.5	...	...	...	...	...	...
With other brain or nervous diseases	4.8	...	9.1	5.6	12.8	1.6	6.1	5.4	4.9	6.6	1.4	3.3	2.8	...	...	...
Alcoholic	38.5	...	50.0	44.0	51.3	43.8	41.6	41.7	39.0	36.8	24.4	31.3	37.8	25.0	12.5	...
Due to drugs and other exogenous toxins	43.2	...	18.2	50.0	38.1	35.7	49.2	43.0	63.0	39.4	38.5	40.0	64.3	66.7	100.0	...
With pellagra	14.7	...	22.2	18.8	20.5	8.2	19.7	9.0	23.6	8.2	19.4	11.1	...	...	...	...
With other somatic diseases	23.3	...	25.4	31.3	38.3	25.2	26.7	30.0	15.9	18.2	14.4	14.0	11.0	11.1	...	...
Manic-depressive	35.4	30.8	41.6	43.3	36.7	35.3	37.8	35.8	33.8	31.9	31.9	31.2	27.3	29.8	40.0	20.0
Involution melancholia	15.9	...	...	27.3	7.7	30.4	30.9	14.5	16.4	15.1	15.1	16.0	14.1	17.9	6.7	...
Dementia præcox	6.4	14.3	8.2	7.8	6.2	6.1	6.1	5.9	4.7	5.3	5.3	5.7	4.9	7.5	...	6.7
Paranoia or paranoid conditions	7.9	...	20.0	12.5	8.2	8.1	9.1	10.0	7.1	7.3	7.7	5.4	5.6	6.3	6.7	...
Epileptic	5.2	1.9	4.6	3.9	4.7	4.4	4.8	7.4	8.4	8.7	9.4	5.5	2.6	...	...	...
Psychoneuroses and neuroses	13.5	23.5	25.2	12.2	7.3	11.2	15.9	21.0	15.7	24.1	20.0	12.2	9.1	37.5	...	...
With psychopathic personality	21.2	12.5	13.2	20.3	25.7	27.6	30.7	18.1	19.1	18.2	16.1	6.7	14.3	33.3	...	...
With mental deficiency	10.9	...	9.9	16.1	11.6	12.0	11.1	13.0	6.4	8.2	10.0	4.3	...	12.5	...	...
Undiagnosed psychoses	10.9	5.1	13.0	12.3	12.1	11.7	12.5	12.1	10.9	9.8	9.6	11.9	5.8	2.7	3.0	...
Without psychosis	5.6	0.5	0.8	3.3	6.9	5.4	7.4	6.1	7.3	6.2	5.9	3.1	7.6	4.7	...	...
Unascertained	4.9	...	20.0	7.4	...	6.9	4.5	6.9	...	...	12.5	15.0	10.0	...	...	...
Total	13.5	4.8	13.4	15.2	14.1	14.4	16.7	16.8	15.9	15.6	13.5	10.7	6.9	3.9	2.5	0.3

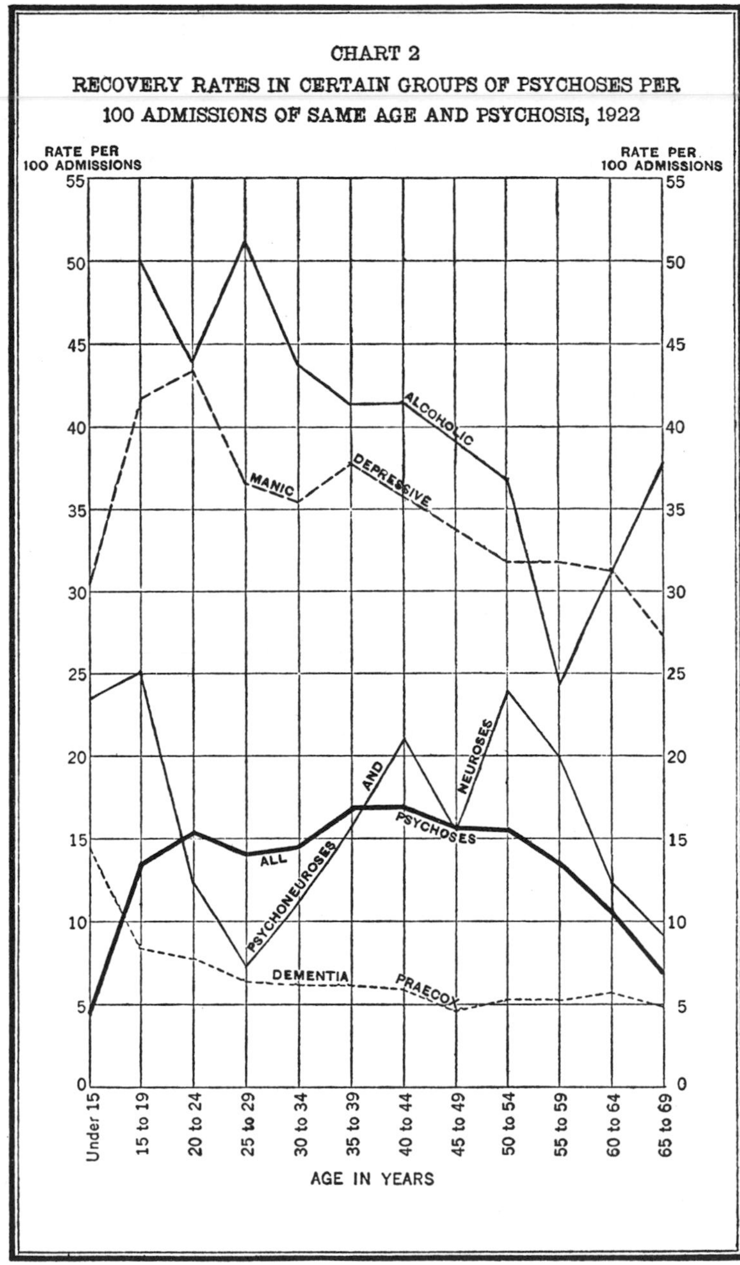
CHART 2
RECOVERY RATES IN CERTAIN GROUPS OF PSYCHOSES PER 100 ADMISSIONS OF SAME AGE AND PSYCHOSIS, 1922
RATE PER 100 ADMISSIONS
RATE PER 100 ADMISSIONS
55
50
45
40
35
30
25
20
15
10
5
0
ALCOHOLIC
MANIC
DEPRESSIVE
PSYCHONEUROSES
AND
NEUROSES
ALL
PSYCHOSES
DEMENTIA
PRAECOX
Under 15
15 to 19
20 to 24
25 to 29
30 to 34
35 to 39
40 to 44
45 to 49
50 to 54
55 to 59
60 to 64
65 to 69
AGE IN YEARS

In the separate psychoses the variation in recovery rates in the several age groups is much greater. In certain psychoses the number of recovered cases, when separated by age periods, is too small to furnish a satisfactory basis for rates; but in some of the larger groups age appears to be a factor of considerable importance in influencing recovery. In the alcoholic psychoses, the recovery rate is much higher in the age groups below 45 years than in the groups above that age. In the manic-depressive psychoses the recovery rate is highest among patients 15 to 25 years of age, although there continues to be a high rate of recoveries in this group in every age period up to 80 years.

Females have a higher recovery rate than males in each age group up to 65 years. The highest recovery rate among the females occurs in the age group 35 to 39 years, while the highest rate among the males occurs in the group 40 to 44 years.

TABLE 5. PER CENT DISTRIBUTION OF PATIENTS DISCHARGED AS RECOVERED FROM HOSPITALS FOR MENTAL DISEASE DURING 1922, BY PSYCHOSIS* AND LENGTH OF HOSPITAL RESIDENCE**

Psychoses	Total	Under 4 months	4 to 6 months	7 to 11 months	1 year	2 years	3 years	4 years	5 years and over
Alcoholic	100.0	72.4	11.4	7.0	5.2	1.0	0.7	0.6	1.7
Due to drugs and other exogenous toxins ..	100.0	68.9	13.8	6.0	7.5	1.2	0.6	0.6	1.5
With other somatic diseases	100.0	62.1	16.1	13.5	4.1	1.3	1.5	...	1.3
Manic-depressive	100.0	35.8	19.6	14.8	15.5	5.2	3.0	1.8	4.2
Involution melancholia	100.0	33.0	21.2	13.3	16.2	3.2	3.8	1.8	7.4
Dementia præcox	100.0	28.8	22.1	17.0	15.0	6.0	3.0	1.6	6.4
Paranoia or paranoid conditions	100.0	43.7	14.8	13.7	10.9	4.9	2.7	...	9.3
Epileptic psychoses...	100.0	47.8	12.2	13.0	13.0	4.3	2.6	0.9	6.1
Psychoneuroses and neuroses	100.0	56.2	18.4	10.2	9.6	2.0	1.6	0.2	1.6
With psychopathic personality	100.0	34.7	15.8	15.8	18.5	3.5	1.9	3.9	5.8
With mental deficiency	100.0	36.1	17.1	14.3	16.3	5.2	2.4	2.8	6.0
Undiagnosed psychoses	100.0	56.5	15.3	9.7	8.5	3.1	1.7	0.4	4.7
Without psychosis ..	100.0	77.3	10.1	4.2	5.6	1.4	0.6	0.3	0.3
Total patients	100.0	44.3	17.9	13.2	12.8	4.1	2.4	1.4	4.0

*Per cents not shown for psychoses with less than 100 recovered cases.

**The percentages of cases the length of whose hospital residence was unascertained are omitted.

The per cent distribution of patients discharged as recovered classified by length of hospital residence is shown for the larger groups of psychoses in Table 5. Most recoveries occur during the early periods of hospital life, 44.3 per cent occurring during the first four months of hospital life, and 75.4 per cent within the first year. Recovery is naturally more rapid in some forms of mental disease than in others. In the alcoholic group 72.4 per cent, and in

TABLE 6. PER CENT DISTRIBUTION OF PATIENTS DISCHARGED AS IMPROVED FROM HOSPITALS FOR MENTAL DISEASE DURING 1922, BY PSYCHOSIS* AND LENGTH OF HOSPITAL RESIDENCE**

Psychoses	Total	Under 4 months	4 to 6 months	7 to 11 months	1 year	2 years	3 years	4 years	5 years and over
Senile	100.0	49.0	15.1	10.9	11.8	4.3	2.4	2.1	4.5
With cerebral arterio-sclerosis	100.0	53.1	18.8	10.9	12.0	1.4	0.9	1.2	1.7
General paralysis	100.0	45.8	17.5	14.4	12.6	4.3	3.3	0.6	1.6
With cerebral syphilis	100.0	45.7	20.0	14.3	13.9	3.3	0.8	1.2	0.8
With other brain or nervous diseases	100.0	65.3	9.3	8.7	9.3	1.3	1.3	1.3	3.3
Alcoholic	100.0	66.0	7.4	7.7	8.1	3.1	2.7	1.0	4.0
Due to drugs and other exogenous toxins	100.0	74.9	8.9	5.5	5.5	2.2	0.4	0.4	2.2
With pellagra	100.0	52.8	13.6	15.2	12.0	3.2	2.4	...	0.8
With other somatic diseases	100.0	62.3	15.2	8.4	7.9	3.1	1.5	0.4	1.1
Manic-depressive	100.0	41.6	16.5	13.6	13.5	5.4	2.7	1.6	5.1
Involution melancholia	100.0	40.8	15.6	14.3	14.3	4.2	2.7	2.0	6.1
Dementia præcox	100.0	30.7	16.2	15.5	16.8	6.8	4.0	2.3	7.7
Paranoia or paranoid conditions	100.0	40.5	13.3	10.0	14.7	5.5	3.1	3.1	9.9
Epileptic psychoses	100.0	44.4	11.6	9.6	17.8	4.9	3.4	1.8	6.3
Psychoneuroses and neuroses	100.0	54.5	16.2	15.5	10.3	1.6	0.6	0.4	0.7
With psychopathic personality	100.0	42.9	17.5	9.7	16.1	5.9	2.1	2.1	3.1
With mental deficiency	100.0	30.2	14.9	16.1	17.2	7.3	3.3	1.6	9.5
Undiagnosed psychoses	100.0	54.6	12.6	9.7	10.4	3.7	1.8	1.6	5.7
Without psychosis	100.0	65.1	10.7	10.7	7.4	2.5	1.4	0.8	1.4
Total patients	100.0	43.4	15.3	13.2	13.6	4.8	2.7	1.6	5.2

*Per cents not shown for psychoses with less than 100 improved cases.

**The percentages of cases the length of whose hospital residence was unascertained are omitted.

the drug group 68.9 per cent, of the recoveries occurred within four months of admission. In the manic-depressive group 35.8 per cent of the recoveries occurred within four months of hospital life, 19.6 per cent additional occurred in the period of 4 to 6 months, and 14.8 per cent additional in the period of 7 to 11 months. In the involution melancholia, dementia præcox, paranoid, epileptic, psychopathic personality, and mental deficiency groups a considerable percentage of recoveries occur after a hospital residence of five years or more.

Table 6 gives the per cent distribution of the patients discharged as improved, classified by psychosis and length of hospital residence. It is noteworthy that 71.9 per cent of all cases discharged as improved had a hospital residence of less than one year, and that 43.4 per cent had a hospital residence of less than four months. In nearly all the clinical groups there was a high percentage of improved cases discharged within four months from the time of admission.

Deaths

Patients leave institutions for mental disease either by discharge or death. Transfers, of course, are frequently made from one institution for mental disease to another in the same state; while such transfers reduce the population of the institution from which they go, they do not change the population of the institutions as a whole. They are, therefore, not given special consideration in this discussion.

Of the 25,656 deaths reported by the hospitals for mental disease in 1922, individual schedules were received for 25,436, of whom 14,769 were males and 10,667 females. The general death rate per 1,000 patients under treatment was 74.3. The rate for males was 80.1 and for females 67.4. The lower death rate of female patients corresponds in a measure to the lower death rate of females in the general population, but in the institutions the difference in death rate in the two sexes is greater, due principally to the excess of males in the general paralysis group, in which the death rate is very high. Comparing deaths with admissions, we find that in 1922 the number of deaths was 27.7 per cent of the number of total admissions. As the number of discharges, excluding deaths and

TABLE 7. COMPARISON OF DEATHS IN HOSPITALS FOR MENTAL DISEASE BY STATES DURING 1922 AND 1910, WITH RATES PER 1,000 OF TOTAL UNDER TREATMENT EACH YEAR

States	1922						1910					
	Number of deaths			Per 1,000 under treatment			Number of deaths			Per 1,000 under treatment		
	M.	F.	T.	M.	F.	T.	M.	F.	T.	M.	F.	T.
Alabama	160	101	261	93.6	56.2	77.4	157	170	327	112.7	120.6	116.7
Arizona	41	10	51	90.3	53.2	79.4	36	8	44	105.9	92.0	103.0
Arkansas	181	87	268	104.4	61.9	85.4	68	50	118	104.6	76.2	90.4
California ...	772	467	1,239	78.4	72.0	75.8	414	194	608	82.4	64.6	75.7
Colorado	130	75	205	90.3	65.2	79.2	82	33	115	86.4	51.8	72.5
Connecticut ..	256	168	424	77.1	51.6	64.5	172	139	311	78.9	59.1	68.6
Delaware ...	20	17	37	59.9	59.9	59.9	23	25	48	77.4	98.0	87.0
District of Columbia ..	197	70	267	56.3	58.7	56.9	206	73	279	79.4	83.4	80.4
Florida	144	81	225	105.6	78.2	93.8	76	42	118	130.6	84.7	109.5
Georgia	152	149	301	55.6	55.6	55.6	241	214	455	116.1	106.0	111.2
Idaho	46	23	69	95.0	81.0	89.8	23	10	33	65.7	60.6	64.1
Illinois	1,184	766	1,950	84.2	67.8	76.9	784	568	1,352	89.3	77.2	83.8
Indiana	267	196	463	63.9	55.2	59.9	277	158	435	99.7	57.3	78.5
Iowa	344	204	548	68.1	52.5	61.3	308	188	496	84.9	61.6	74.3
Kansas	181	95	276	78.4	49.5	65.3	195	91	286	91.2	60.7	78.6
Kentucky	286	224	510	84.0	82.4	83.3	252	172	424	97.0	84.6	91.6
Louisiana ...	123	101	224	56.7	47.6	52.2	95	91	186	74.8	70.5	72.7
Maine	108	72	180	88.4	66.6	78.2	83	83	166	92.8	111.9	101.5
Maryland	271	197	468	73.4	66.5	70.3	167	154	321	80.7	73.1	76.8
Massachusetts	797	762	1,559	73.9	71.0	72.4	632	519	1,151	87.8	69.6	78.5
Michigan	520	319	839	81.2	61.7	72.5	431	268	699	91.6	70.5	82.2
Minnesota ...	343	206	549	71.2	59.2	66.2	251	134	385	73.1	55.5	65.8
Mississippi ...	150	133	283	72.6	77.5	74.8	111	126	237	89.5	93.3	91.5
Missouri	542	356	898	89.8	66.9	79.0	402	283	685	93.9	74.7	84.9
Nebraska	175	97	272	83.9	60.6	73.8	116	58	174	86.1	60.2	75.3
Nevada	7	6	13	41.7	73.2	52.0	13	8	21	63.7	98.8	73.7
New Hampshire	101	60	161	111.6	71.3	92.2	80	66	146	131.4	112.2	122.0
New Jersey .	532	485	1,017	96.2	83.4	89.6	344	258	602	93.6	67.7	80.4
New Mexico ..	21	24	45	71.2	118.8	90.5	32	7	39	177.8	66.0	136.4
New York ...	2,078	1,945	4,023	82.9	75.1	78.9	1,499	1,244	2,743	81.2	63.9	72.4
No. Carolina..	145	153	298	68.9	57.3	62.4	115	99	214	85.2	53.5	66.9
No. Dakota...	53	33	86	56.5	57.8	57.0	39	14	53	80.6	54.5	71.5
Ohio	861	573	1,434	92.5	72.7	83.4	713	434	1,147	96.5	69.9	84.4
Oklahoma	200	108	308	92.4	66.2	81.1	94	61	155	92.7	85.9	89.9
Oregon	190	109	299	85.4	92.1	87.8	119	34	153	84.5	55.5	75.7
Pennsylvania..	1,154	878	2,032	85.4	72.4	79.2	835	702	1,537	84.1	79.6	82.0
Rhode Island.	121	74	195	107.5	75.4	92.5	76	60	136	86.5	76.8	81.9
So. Carolina..	186	115	301	112.0	72.8	92.9	150	147	297	144.5	129.4	136.6
So. Dakota ..	65	29	94	73.8	46.6	62.5	54	27	81	85.0	69.8	79.3
Tennessee ...	153	142	295	61.8	61.7	61.8	119	126	245	78.1	84.2	81.2
Texas	297	201	498	69.7	49.1	59.6	210	157	367	77.5	63.8	70.9
Utah	38	24	62	76.8	55.0	66.6	19	18	37	83.7	87.4	85.5
Vermont	79	68	147	92.9	88.5	90.9	62	48	110	91.4	83.5	87.8
Virginia	249	176	425	72.7	57.4	65.5	239	182	421	103.7	79.5	91.6
Washington ..	257	106	363	83.1	59.0	74.3	168	52	220	92.9	59.8	82.2
West Virginia..	172	104	276	111.1	78.7	96.2	98	76	174	85.7	74.1	80.3
Wisconsin ...	398	273	671	59.2	55.7	57.7	299	191	490	63.7	54.5	59.8
Wyoming ...	22	5	27	58.5	41.3	54.3	6	5	11	48.8	73.5	57.6
Total	14,769	10,667	25,436	80.1	67.4	74.3	11,045	7,879	18,924	87.7	71.6	80.2

transfers, was 58.4 per cent of the number of admissions, it is evident that patients are entering institutions for mental disease considerably faster than they are leaving.

Table 7 compares death rates per 1,000 under treatment in hospitals for mental disease in 1910 and 1922, the data being taken from the Federal Census report of the respective years. In 1910 the general death rate of patients was 80.2, the rate for males 87.7, and for females 71.6. The lower death rate in 1922 confirms the general belief that the care of patients with mental disease has improved considerably since 1910. While the trend of death rates in institutions for mental disease in most states has gone down with the general trend, an increase in death rate in several states in 1922 is noted. For example, the death rate among patients in Rhode Island in 1910 was 81.9 and in 1922, 92.5; in New York in 1910, 72.4 and in 1922, 78.9; in New Jersey in 1910, 80.4 and in 1922, 89.6. Death rates in the several states are influenced by many factors, the most important of which are the age and type of mental disease of the patients under treatment.

Death rates for the several psychotic groups are shown by sex in Table 8. A remarkably wide range of death rates is seen in the various psychoses, the highest rate—305.9—being found in the cerebral arteriosclerotic group and the lowest rate—14.4—in the psychoneuroses and neuroses group. High death rates are found in the so-called organic groups and the somatic disease group and comparatively low rates in the toxic and functional groups. Females have lower death rates than males in all of the organic groups except that of psychoses with other brain or nervous diseases, and in the manic-depressive, involution melancholia, and epileptic groups. Males have lower death rates in the alcoholic, drug, dementia præcox, paranoid, and psychoneuroses and neuroses groups. No adequate explanation can be made for these marked differences in death rates among patients of the two sexes.

The influence of the various classes of disease in causing deaths of patients in the several clinical groups is shown by Table 9. The death rate in all clinical groups from general diseases was 13.9; from diseases of the nervous system, 26.7; from diseases of the circulatory system, 18.0; from diseases of the respiratory system, 5.9; from diseases of the digestive system, 2.1; from diseases of the genito-urinary system, 4.1; and from violence, 1.3. The rates from the several causes in the various groups of psychoses bear little resemblance to the general average rate. The rates in each group are also unlike those of any other.

TABLE 8. PATIENTS DYING IN HOSPITALS FOR MENTAL DISEASE DURING 1922, CLASSIFIED BY PSYCHOSIS, WITH RATES PER 1,000 OF TOTAL UNDER TREATMENT DURING THE YEAR WITH SAME PSYCHOSIS

Psychoses	Number of deaths			Per 1,000 under treatment		
	Males	Females	Total	Males	Females	Total
Traumatic	33	9	42	51.6	101.1	57.7
Senile	2,643	2,431	5,074	280.7	221.4	248.7
With cerebral arteriosclerosis	1,530	820	2,350	319.1	284.0	305.9
General paralysis	3,816	869	4,685	304.0	261.4	295.0
With cerebral syphilis	278	101	379	157.5	120.0	145.4
With Huntington's chorea	35	35	70	177.7	156.3	166.3
With brain tumor	19	14	33	275.4	274.5	275.0
With other brain or nervous diseases	169	117	286	171.2	175.1	172.8
Alcoholic	331	82	413	37.2	56.1	39.9
Due to drugs and other exogenous toxins	34	33	67	43.4	62.4	51.1
With pellagra	76	158	234	254.2	235.8	241.5
With other somatic diseases	326	366	692	217.2	164.0	185.4
Manic-depressive	1,164	1,481	2,645	49.5	46.5	47.7
Involution melancholia	239	381	620	97.7	71.9	80.0
Dementia præcox	1,930	2,018	3,948	27.8	33.5	30.5
Paranoia or paranoid conditions	175	227	402	26.8	31.3	29.2
Epileptic	606	413	1,019	96.0	84.8	91.1
Psychoneuroses and neuroses	33	52	85	9.4	21.9	14.4
With psychopathic personality	49	29	78	21.1	19.0	20.3
With mental deficiency	213	201	414	29.1	32.4	30.6
Undiagnosed psychoses	668	561	1,229	66.9	67.7	67.3
Without psychosis	346	223	569	34.2	40.3	36.4
Unascertained	56	46	102	56.3	57.9	57.0
Total	14,769	10,667	25,436	80.1	67.4	74.3

TABLE 9. DEATH RATES PER 1,000 UNDER TREATMENT FROM THE VARIOUS CLASSES OF DISEASES OF PATIENTS IN HOSPITALS FOR MENTAL DISEASE DURING 1922, BY PSYCHOSES

Psychoses	Total	General diseases	Diseases of nervous system	Diseases of circulatory system	Diseases of respiratory system	Diseases of digestive system	Diseases of the genito-urinary system	Diseases of the skin	Violence	All other causes	Unascertained
Traumatic	57.7	5.5	13.7	13.7	6.9	1.4	4.1	...	11.0	1.4	...
Senile	248.7	17.0	34.8	111.3	30.0	5.9	18.7	1.4	2.7	26.8	0.1
With cerebral arteriosclerosis	305.9	10.2	67.6	185.8	24.1	1.0	16.3	...	1.0	...	...
General paralysis	295.0	1.3	291.1	0.4	0.3	...	0.1	...	1.8	...	...
With cerebral syphilis	145.4	106.6	34.5	2.3	...	...	0.4	...	1.5	...	...
With Huntington's chorea	166.3	19.0	104.5	14.3	9.5	9.5	9.5	...	...	...	...
With brain tumor	275.0	8.3	250.0	8.3	...	...	...	...	8.3	...	...
With other brain or nervous diseases	172.8	27.2	105.1	21.8	10.3	2.4	4.8	...	0.6	0.6	...
Alcoholic	39.9	16.1	5.0	7.5	4.4	1.9	3.8	...	1.1	...	...
Due to drugs and other exogenous toxins	51.1	17.5	6.1	16.0	2.3	...	6.9	...	2.3	...	...
With pellagra	241.5	239.4	...	...	...	...	1.0	...	1.0	...	...
With other somatic diseases	185.4	67.0	19.6	40.7	13.1	7.2	32.7	...	3.1	2.4	0.5
Manic-depressive	47.7	11.0	14.7	9.2	4.4	2.5	3.7	0.1	2.0	0.1	...
Involution melancholia	80.0	12.7	17.8	22.7	9.7	5.3	6.8	0.4	4.1	0.5	...
Dementia præcox	30.5	13.0	4.8	5.5	2.9	1.6	1.7	0.1	0.7	0.2	*
Paranoia or paranoid conditions	29.2	7.5	4.4	9.2	3.0	1.4	2.9	0.2	0.5	...	0.1
Epileptic	91.1	11.7	63.2	4.9	6.5	1.0	2.1	0.1	1.4	0.1	...
Psychoneuroses and neuroses	14.4	3.9	2.5	2.5	1.4	0.7	1.2	...	2.0	...	0.2
With psychopathic personality	20.3	7.3	3.1	2.9	2.9	2.1	1.0	0.3	0.8	...	...
With mental deficiency	30.6	11.3	4.5	6.1	3.8	2.4	1.7	...	0.5	0.1	0.1
Undiagnosed psychoses	67.3	14.1	13.8	17.9	7.8	2.8	5.0	0.4	1.9	0.9	2.6
Without psychosis	36.4	12.2	7.4	7.9	4.3	1.2	2.3	0.1	0.6	0.3	0.2
Unascertained	57.0	7.8	5.6	7.3	7.8	3.4	3.9	1.1	1.1	1.1	17.9
Total	74.3	13.9	26.7	18.0	5.9	2.1	4.1	0.2	1.3	1.8	0.3

*Less than one-tenth of 1 per 1,000.

Death rates among males and females from principal diseases were as follows:

Diseases	Rates per 1,000 under treatment Males	Females	Total
Tuberculosis of lungs	6.6	8.1	7.3
Cancer	1.1	1.9	1.5
Apoplexy	5.5	4.8	5.2
General paralysis	21.7	6.0	14.4
Bronchopneumonia	2.7	3.0	2.8
Lobar pneumonia	2.2	2.2	2.2
Diarrhea and enteritis	0.6	1.3	0.9
Nephritis, all forms	3.8	4.0	3.9
Suicide	0.8	0.5	0.7
All other cases	35.3	35.5	35.4

The most striking difference shown in this tabulation is the greater prevalence of general paralysis among males.

The age distribution of the patients dying in institutions for mental disease is shown in Table 10 below. The number of deaths among males exceeds those among females in each period, although the percentages of deaths among females are greater than those among males in the age groups under 35 years and those of 65 years and over.

TABLE 10. AGE DISTRIBUTION OF PATIENTS DYING IN HOSPITALS FOR MENTAL DISEASE DURING 1922

Age groups	Number of deaths			Per cent of total		
	Males	Females	Total	Males	Females	Total
Under 20 years	134	111	245	0.9	1.0	1.0
20 to 24 years	326	274	600	2.2	2.6	2.4
25 to 29 years	504	492	996	3.4	4.6	3.9
30 to 34 years	856	652	1,508	5.8	6.1	5.9
35 to 39 years	1,275	775	2,050	8.6	7.3	8.1
40 to 44 years	1,403	847	2,250	9.5	7.9	8.8
45 to 49 years	1,285	906	2,191	8.7	8.5	8.6
50 to 54 years	1,285	862	2,147	8.7	8.1	8.4
55 to 59 years	1,266	809	2,075	8.6	7.6	8.2
60 to 64 years	1,430	938	2,368	9.7	8.8	9.3
65 years and over	4,826	3,897	8,723	32.7	36.5	34.3
Unascertained	179	104	283	1.2	1.0	1.1
Total	14,769	10,667	25,436	100.0	100.0	100.0

Only 7.3 per cent of the patients dying were under 30 years and only 1.0 per cent under 20 years of age; 32.7 per cent of the males and 36.5 per cent of the females reached 65 years or over.

Death rates per 1,000 under treatment in the several age groups are shown in Table 11. Among the females the death rate rises in each successive age group from 20 years upwards, with the exception of group 30 to 34 years. Among the males there is a slight fall in the rate in the age period 25 to 29 years, but a steady rise in the succeeding groups. The death rate among females is higher than among males in the age groups under 35 years and much lower in the remaining age groups. The fatal effects of general paralysis account for a large part of the excessive death rates among males in age periods above 40 years.

TABLE 11. DEATH RATES PER 1,000 UNDER TREATMENT BY AGE GROUPS AMONG PATIENTS IN INSTITUTIONS FOR MENTAL DISEASE IN THE UNITED STATES, 1922

Age groups	Males	Females	Total
Under 20 years	35.3	37.4	36.2
20 to 24 years	32.2	44.1	36.7
25 to 29 years	30.2	44.2	35.8
30 to 34 years	42.1	43.5	42.7
35 to 39 years	56.9	44.4	51.4
40 to 44 years	65.3	46.4	56.6
45 to 49 years	66.2	50.0	58.4
50 to 54 years	74.6	50.7	62.7
55 to 59 years	87.8	58.2	73.2
60 to 64 years	112.7	74.9	93.9
65 years and over	214.3	165.1	189.1
Total	80.1	67.4	74.3

That patients with mental disease have a much higher death rate at all ages than the general population is seen by comparing the foregoing rates with those compiled by the Federal Census Bureau for the registration area of the United States in 1920. (See Table 12.)

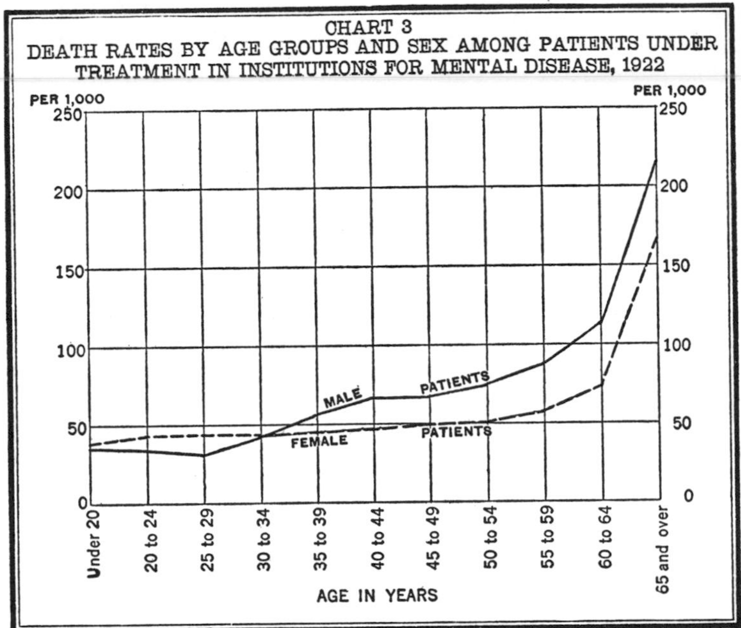

TABLE 12. DEATH RATES PER 1,000 BY AGE GROUPS AMONG THE GENERAL POPULATION OF THE REGISTRATION AREA OF THE UNITED STATES, 1920*

Age groups	Males	Females	Total
15 to 19 years	4.2	4.0	4.1
20 to 24 years	5.4	6.0	5.7
25 to 34 years	6.5	7.2	6.9
35 to 44 years	8.4	8.1	8.3
45 to 54 years	12.6	11.8	12.2
55 to 64 years	24.9	22.8	23.9
65 to 74 years	54.7	50.7	52.7
75 years and over	137.4	133.0	135.1
Total	13.5	12.7	13.1

*Mortality Rates, 1910-1920. Federal Census Report, p. 428.

The average age at death of all patients who died in institutions for mental disease in 1922 was found to be 55.3. This average age is nearly the same as that of the persons dying in the general population, but it must be remembered that patients with mental disease are in the main an adult group. In the separate groups of psychoses the average age at death varies from 42.9 years in the epileptic group to 74.1 years in the senile group. Among general paralysis patients the average age at death was found to be 45.2 years, and among dementia præcox patients, 46.5. (See Table 13.)

Table 13. Average Age at Death of Patients Dying in Hospitals for Mental Disease During 1922, Classified by Psychosis

Psychoses	Average age at death
Traumatic	53.2
Senile	74.1
With cerebral arteriosclerosis	67.4
General paralysis	45.2
With cerebral syphilis	47.8
With Huntington's chorea	53.4
With brain tumor	45.8
With other brain or nervous diseases	51.5
Alcoholic	55.8
Due to drugs and other exogenous toxins	54.3
With pellagra	43.7
With other somatic diseases	48.2
Manic-depressive	50.8
Involution melancholia	58.3
Dementia præcox	46.5
Paranoia or paranoid conditions	61.4
Epileptic	42.9
Psychoneuroses and neuroses	46.3
With psychopathic personality	44.9
With mental deficiency	45.9
Undiagnosed	55.1
Without psychosis	47.1
Unascertained	59.8
Total	55.3

Table 14 shows the per cent distribution of hospital life periods of patients dying in institutions in 1922 classified by psychosis.

TABLE 14. PER CENT DISTRIBUTION BY LENGTH OF HOSPITAL RESIDENCE OF PATIENTS DYING DURING 1922, CLASSIFIED BY PSYCHOSIS*

Psychoses	** Total	Under 1 month	1 month	2 months	3 months	4 months	5 months	6 months	7 to 11 months	1 year	2 years	3 years	4 years	5 to 9 years	10 years and over
Senile	100.0	18.0	9.4	6.3	5.4	4.3	3.4	2.6	10.5	13.0	7.2	4.6	3.1	7.1	5.1
With cerebral arterio-sclerosis	100.0	26.7	11.4	6.8	4.5	4.7	3.5	3.2	9.6	13.1	5.3	2.9	2.0	3.8	2.4
General paralysis	100.0	13.1	8.9	6.2	5.4	4.7	3.6	3.8	12.8	20.8	9.6	4.4	2.3	3.5	0.8
With cerebral syphilis	100.0	17.9	7.4	7.9	6.3	4.7	4.5	2.4	11.6	15.0	6.9	4.2	4.0	4.0	3.2
With other brain or nervous diseases	100.0	30.4	11.2	5.9	4.5	2.8	2.8	1.7	8.4	10.1	4.2	5.2	1.4	6.6	4.5
Alcoholic	100.0	14.0	3.4	2.7	2.2	0.7	1.0	0.7	4.1	6.5	1.5	4.8	6.5	20.8	31.0
With pellagra	100.0	29.9	18.4	11.1	3.4	4.3	3.0	3.8	7.7	6.8	3.4	1.7	2.6	1.7	2.1
With other somatic diseases	100.0	53.2	12.4	5.6	3.8	3.3	2.3	1.3	5.6	3.9	1.6	1.4	1.2	3.0	1.3
Manic-depressive	100.0	19.6	5.6	3.1	2.9	2.2	2.1	1.9	7.1	8.8	6.0	4.0	3.4	12.2	21.1
Involution melancholia	100.0	11.8	9.0	6.6	5.8	4.7	1.5	1.6	7.4	10.6	6.3	2.1	2.7	9.7	20.2
Dementia præcox	100.0	4.2	2.0	1.4	1.2	1.0	0.7	1.0	4.1	8.2	7.1	5.4	5.3	17.4	41.1
Paranoia or paranoid conditions	100.0	2.5	3.5	2.5	1.2	1.0	0.7	1.2	2.5	5.5	5.5	4.7	4.2	16.9	48.0
Epileptic	100.0	5.7	2.6	2.6	2.1	1.5	1.6	1.1	7.0	10.8	8.6	6.4	5.9	21.3	23.0
With mental deficiency	100.0	2.7	1.9	1.9	2.4	1.4	1.0	1.0	6.8	13.3	8.2	8.2	4.8	18.1	28.3
Undiagnosed	100.0	28.9	6.3	3.9	2.8	1.9	1.3	1.5	5.9	6.7	3.3	2.8	1.7	7.8	24.9
Without psychosis	100.0	12.3	7.9	3.0	2.6	2.3	2.3	1.6	4.7	12.5	8.1	7.0	4.6	13.4	17.8
Unascertained	100.0	11.8	2.9	8.8	3.9	1.0	1.0	1.0	3.9	8.8	2.9	2.9	2.0	8.8	36.3
Total patients	100.0	16.3	7.2	4.7	3.8	3.2	2.5	2.2	8.4	12.2	6.9	4.4	3.3	9.5	15.2

*Per cent not shown for groups of psychoses with less than 100 patients.

**The percentages of cases the length of whose hospital residence was unascertained are omitted.

It is noteworthy that the hospital life of 16.3 per cent of the patients who died was less than one month; 23.5 per cent had a hospital life of less than two months; and 48.3 per cent had a hospital life of less than one year. On the other hand 15.2 per cent had been in the institutions 10 years or more. The patients of each group of psychoses have a characteristic distribution of hospital life periods. The forms of mental disease accompanied by acute physical diseases which terminate fatally naturally are represented by a comparatively brief period of hospital life. For example, 53.2 per cent of the patients in the group psychoses with other somatic diseases who died in the hospitals had a hospital life of less than one month. Other groups with a high percentage of deaths occurring within one month of hospital life are general paralysis, psychoses with other brain or nervous diseases, psychoses with pellagra, and undiagnosed psychoses. The groups in which large percentages of deaths occurred after a hospital life of 10 years or more are alcoholic, dementia præcox, paranoia or paranoid conditions, and psychoses with mental deficiency.

Although the scope of this chapter will not permit a detailed discussion of the outcome of each form of mental disease, the data presented in the several tables will throw considerable light on the matter. It will be evident to any one who seriously considers the matter that both general and detailed data are necessary to a clear understanding of the results of institutional treatment of mental disease.

CHAPTER IV

Economic Loss to New York State and the United States on Account of Mental Disease, 1931*†

The economic burden due to mental disease has been called to the attention of the people of New York State during the past eight years by three campaigns on behalf of proposals for bond issues for the building of state institutions. The proposals, all of which were approved by the voters, provided, in 1923, for a bond issue of $50,000,000 for state hospitals and other institutions; in 1925, for a bond issue of $100,000,000 for state institutions and other improvements, to be made available at the rate of $10,000,000 a year; and in 1930, for a bond issue of $50,000,000 for state hospitals and state prisons. About $90,000,000 of the proceeds of these bond issues has been or will be devoted to the construction of hospitals for patients with mental disease. Another phase of the burden was emphasized by the appropriation, in 1931, of nearly $24,000,000 for the maintenance of patients with mental disease in the hospitals of the New York State Department of Mental Hygiene.

New light on the economic loss due to mental disease was made available in 1930 by the publication of an important book, *The Money Value of Man,* by Drs. Dublin and Lotka of the Metropolitan Life Insurance Company. Prior to the publication of this study, there was no authoritative work to which one could turn for information concerning the economic value of persons with varying earning capacity at different age periods.

The present review of economic loss on account of mental disease supplements two previous papers by the author, one dealing with the economic loss to the state of New York on account of insanity in 1911, the other with the economic loss on account of hospital cases of mental disease and associated physical disorders in New York State in 1928. So far as known, no similar studies have been made. In dealing with the topic before us, we shall first attempt an analysis of the economic loss to New York State on account of mental

*Read at the Annual Meeting of the American Statistical Association, Washington, D. C., December 30, 1931.

†The loss from year to year will vary with the number of patients cared for and with the cost of maintenance and of hospital construction. The method used here may be applied to any similar data in calculating the annual loss to a state or country on account of mental disease.

disease in 1931 and shall then apply the results obtained in making estimates for the country as a whole. We have limited our study to hospital cases of mental disease. We recognize that the loss due to mild cases of mental disease cared for outside of state hospitals and licensed institutions is quite large, but as little is known concerning the number of such cases or the duration or severity of their illnesses, any estimate of such loss would be merely an unsupported guess. We deem it better to heed psychiatric counsel and hold fast to reality so far as possible.

Physical disorders play a prominent part in the causation and prolongation of mental disorders. In several of the groups of psychoses, physical and psychic elements are so intertwined that they cannot be separated. In other groups, physical factors play a less conspicuous part. No way has yet been devised of calculating or estimating the relative importance of the two factors. In this study no attempt is made to evaluate physical factors or other causes contributing to mental illnesses.

The economic loss due to hospital cases of mental disease consists of two principal items:

I. The cost of maintenance of patients in hospitals.

II. The loss of earnings due to the disability and premature death of the patients.

The Cost of Maintenance

The cost of maintenance of patients in hospitals comprises three factors:

A. Cost of hospital care and treatment, including medical and nursing services, food, clothing, care of buildings and grounds, and all other items that are essential to the comfort and well-being of patients in a modern hospital.

B. The investment charge, which includes interest on the outlay for the hospital plant and equipment, and an allowance for depreciation and obsolescence.

C. The cost of general administration. In our own hospital system this comprises the expense of conducting the two administrative offices of the State Department of Mental Hygiene, the Psychiatric Institute, the bureau of special examination, the inspection service, the central purchase of supplies, the services for this Department of the Governor, the Legislature, the courts, the Attorney-General, the State Civil Service Commission, the State Department of Public Works, the State Comptroller, the State Department of Agriculture, and the State Pension Commission.

Cost of Hospital Care and Treatment.—Taking up in order the several maintenance factors for the fiscal year ended June 30, 1931, we find that the per capita expenditures for hospital care and treatment in the civil state hospitals was $421.76 and in the two hospitals for the criminal insane, $541.80. The per capita cost for the year in the licensed institutions is not available, but is estimated at $2,000 per capita.

The Annual Investment Charge.—The annual investment charge consists of two parts:

1. The interest on the value of the hospital plant and equipment necessary to house and otherwise care for the patients.
2. The allowance that must be made for depreciation and obsolescence of buildings and equipment.

To compute the interest charge, we have to determine, first, the value of the hospital property that forms the base, and, secondly, the rate per cent.

The valuation of the present State hospital plants cannot be easily determined. Several of the institutions occupy land within city limits that is worth many million dollars. Just how much, no one can say. Likewise the value of the buildings now in use cannot be accurately estimated.

The difficulties of an adequate appraisement or valuation of the several hospital plants being so great, we deemed it better to consider the present per capita cost of the building and equipping of a new hospital. Even this cannot be definitely determined, as no complete State hospital has been built and equipped in recent years. Judging, however, from the cost of the new units at Kings Park, Creedmoor, and Rockland State hospitals, the present average outlay for plant and equipment per patient is approximately $4,000. We have, therefore, used this figure in computing per capita investment charges in both groups of State hospitals. The capital outlay of the licensed institutions per patient is estimated to be $6,000.

Interest rates vary considerably from time to time. The average rate on first mortgages and good bonds in recent years has been about 5 per cent. On account of exemptions from taxation, government, state and municipal bonds bear somewhat lower rates. On a purely economic basis, it seems probable that 5 per cent is a fair average rate, and we have used it in our computations.

The rate per cent to be charged for depreciation and obsolescence varies according to the type of building or other property under consideration. Land favorably situated does not depreciate. Certain types of equipment depreciate from 10 to 25 per cent a year. Buildings of fireproof construction depreciate but little from year to year, but may become obsolescent in from thirty to fifty years. Wooden buildings depreciate much more rapidly. In view of our inability to segregate the values of the land and the various types of buildings and equipment constituting the hospital plants, we have arbitrarily decided to reckon depreciation and obsolescence at 2 per cent per year. This is clearly too high for the land values and too low for equipment values, but probably represents a fair average. Combining interest and depreciation, the annual investment charge would be 7 per cent of the capital outlay, or $280 per year in the State hospitals and $420 per year in licensed institutions.

The Cost of General Administration.—The expenditures of the administrative offices of the department during the fiscal year of 1931 were $352,219.73. As the combined average daily patient population of the institutions in the department was 54,007, the per capita expenditures amounted to $6.52. This figure does not include any State expenditures for pensions or the costs to other State departments of services rendered in connection with the commitment and care of mental patients. The exact amount of such expenditures cannot be determined, but in view of the fact that considerable work is required of the Legislature, the courts, and several State departments, as previously mentioned, it seems probable that the total per capita cost for administration is approximately $10, and we have used this amount in our computations.

The several maintenance costs reckoned in accordance with the methods above described are summarized in Table 1. They amount in the aggregate to $44,913,504.

TABLE 1. EXPENDITURES FOR MAINTENANCE OF PATIENTS IN INSTITUTIONS FOR MENTAL DISEASE IN NEW YORK STATE, FISCAL YEAR ENDED JUNE 30, 1931

	Total	Civil State hospitals (48,464 patients)	State hospitals for criminal insane (1,909 patients)	Licensed institutions (3,634 patients)
Maintenance and operation	$28,742,714	$20,440,339	$1,034,375	$7,268,000
Investment charge	15,630,720	13,569,920	534,520	1,526,280
General administration	540,070	484,640	19,090	36,340
Total	$44,913,504	$34,494,899	$1,587,985	$8,830,620

LOSS OF EARNINGS DUE TO THE DISABILITY AND PREMATURE DEATH OF PATIENTS WITH MENTAL DISEASE

Mental disease causes complete or partial disability for long periods and materially shortens life. About one-half of the patients who enter mental hospitals finally die therein. The average period of hospital life of those who die in the hospitals is between six and seven years. The death rate among patients is several times as high as among the general population of the same age distribution. From 20 to 25 per cent of the first admissions recover, and from 15 to 20 more are discharged as improved. From 5 to 10 per cent are discharged as unimproved or as without psychosis.

It is probable that the loss for the year due to reduced earning power can best be determined by considering only the new cases, or first admissions, entering the hospitals. The loss thus viewed would be the present worth of that portion of the future earnings that is cut off by mental disease. The problem thus considered resolves itself into two parts:

A. Determining the present worth of the net future earnings of an average man and of an average woman at each age of life.

B. Finding the proportion of future earnings that are lost when the patient is admitted to a hospital for mental disease.

Fortunately, we have at hand the book previously mentioned, *The Money Value of a Man,* by Drs. Dublin and Lotka. In this study the authors calculated the present worth of the net future earnings at each age of men of varied earning capacities. The earnings for the several working years were carefully graduated and deductions were made for the cost of maintenance. The net economic values thus calculated of a man with maximum earning capacity of $2,000 are shown for various ages in Table 2. Such a wage-earner probably represents a fair average of the males who become patients in New York State hospitals. It will be noted that the value at birth is given at $7,000; at 10 years of age, as $14,950; at 20, as $23,850; and at 26, $25,200, which is the maximum. At fifty, the value becomes $13,800, and at sixty, $6,700; at seventy-two, it becomes a minus quantity.

TABLE 2. ECONOMIC VALUE OF A MAN WITH MAXIMUM EARNING CAPACITY OF $2,000 AS CALCULATED BY DRS. DUBLIN AND LOTKA

Age (years)	Value	Age (years)	Value
0	$7,000	40	$20,350
10	14,950	50	13,800
20	23,850	60	6,700
30	24,450	70	400

The economic value of an average woman was not calculated in this study, but is assumed by the authors in an earlier study to be half that of a man. We have used such assumption in our computations.

What proportion of the value of a person is lost when he develops mental disease and enters a state or licensed hospital for treatment? Estimates might be made for all first admissions or for each clinical group separately. The latter method gives a better analysis of the loss and was used in our calculations.

After careful consideration of discharges, deaths, and duration of hospital life in each group, we arrived at certain percentages of loss. These are set forth in the third column of Tables 3 and 4.

It will be noted that the percentage of estimated loss of future earnings in general paralysis cases is 75. Prior to the introduction of treatment by malaria and tryparsamide, the percentage of loss of earnings in this group was close to 100.

As a rule the organic cases are past middle life on admission and present a less hopeful picture than the functional cases. The percentage of loss in senile cases is placed at 95, in arteriosclerotic cases at 85, and in alcoholic cases at 50.

Although there are comparatively few recoveries in the dementia præcox group, a large proportion of the cases improve so that they are able to do some productive work. The loss in this group we have estimated at 75 per cent.

Some of the manic-depressive and psychoneurotic cases are restored to full earning power, while others continue in the hospital until removed by death. On the whole, these two groups are perhaps the most hopeful of all, and we have estimated their loss in earnings as only 40 per cent.

The loss in the group with mental deficiency is placed at 10 per cent, as this group has low earning ability previous to admission to a hospital for mental disease.

In preparing Tables 3 and 4, we first classified by years of age the first admissions to all the State hospitals and the committed first admissions to the licensed institutions of each sex and psychosis. We then multiplied the number of patients of each age by the estimated present value of the net future earnings of an average person of same sex and age. The amounts thus derived for each psychosis were added and the totals were entered in Column 2 of the tables. This column represents the net economic value of average persons of the same age and sex as the first admissions of the several clinical groups, Table 3 showing the values for the males and Table 4 the values for the females.

The next step was to multiply the amounts in Column 2 by the respective percentages of loss shown in Column 3. The products in Column 4 of Table 3 show the losses for the males in each group, and the corresponding column in Table 4 shows in like manner the losses for the females.

Tables 3 and 4 take no account of the 1,914 voluntary and physician's cases admitted to licensed institutions, as the psychoses and ages of these cases were not reported. The cases included 1,125 males and 789 females. Assuming that the average economic value of these patients was the same as that found for the cases of same sex shown in Tables 3 and 4—namely, $15,598 for males and $7,629 for females—and assuming also that 40 per cent of such value was lost on account of mental disease, we find the total loss for the male cases of this group to be $7,019,100; for the female cases, $2,407,-712; and for both sexes combined, $9,426,812. Adding this amount to the totals shown in Tables 3 and 4, we find the present worth of the loss of net future earnings of all first admissions to be $84,425,269.

TABLE 3. ESTIMATED LOSS OF NET FUTURE EARNINGS OF MALE FIRST ADMISSIONS TO INSTITUTIONS FOR MENTAL DISEASE IN NEW YORK, FISCAL YEAR ENDED JUNE 30, 1931

Psychoses	First admissions	Estimated net economic value of average persons of same age	Per cent of estimated value lost on admission	Economic loss due to mental disease
Traumatic	90	$1,238,485	50	$619,243
Senile	340	392,745	95	373,108
With cerebral arteriosclerosis	800	3,197,650	85	2,718,003
General paralysis	744	12,667,380	75	9,500,535
With cerebral syphilis	80	1,311,630	60	786,978
With Huntington's chorea	4	38,550	100	38,550
With brain tumor	15	261,045	95	247,993
With other brain or nervous diseases	87	1,732,920	70	1,213,044
Alcoholic	530	8,518,905	50	4,259,453
Due to drugs and other exogenous toxins	17	262,710	50	131,355
With pellagra	1	19,155	70	13,409
With other somatic diseases	57	783,145	40	313,258
Manic-depressive	534	9,999,230	45	4,499,654
Involution melancholia	97	1,040,420	70	728,294
Dementia præcox	1,396	30,756,840	75	23,067,630
Paranoia or paranoid conditions	38	504,155	75	378,116
Epileptic psychoses	105	1,928,108	85	1,638,892
Psychoneuroses and neuroses	69	1,466,395	40	586,558
With psychopathic personality	152	3,191,920	50	1,595,960
With mental deficiency	152	3,092,670	10	309,267
Undiagnosed psychoses	75	1,343,650	60	806,190
Without psychosis	101	1,793,235	40	717,294
Total	5,484	$85,540,943		$54,542,784

TABLE 4. ESTIMATED LOSS OF NET FUTURE EARNINGS OF FEMALE FIRST ADMISSIONS TO INSTITUTIONS FOR MENTAL DISEASE IN NEW YORK, FISCAL YEAR ENDED JUNE 30, 1931

Psychoses	First admissions	Estimated net economic value of average persons of same age	Per cent of estimated value lost on admission	Economic loss due to mental disease
Traumatic	11	$60,830	50	$30,415
Senile	450	291,970	95	277,372
With cerebral arteriosclerosis	602	1,405,535	85	1,194,705
General paralysis	215	1,918,408	75	1,438,806
With cerebral syphilis	26	178,775	60	107,265
With Huntington's chorea	9	72,460	100	72,460
With brain tumor	2	18,113	95	17,207
With other brain or nervous diseases	46	427,525	70	299,268
Alcoholic	105	875,998	50	437,999
Due to drugs and other exogenous toxins	11	91,233	50	45,617
With pellagra	...	....	70	....
With other somatic diseases	126	1,106,508	40	442,603
Manic-depressive	757	7,526,558	45	3,386,951
Involution melancholia	189	1,226,445	70	858,512
Dementia præcox	1,175	11,862,890	75	8,897,168
Paranoia or paranoid conditions	54	370,403	75	277,802
Epileptic psychoses	79	808,970	85	687,625
Psychoneuroses and neuroses	133	1,321,570	40	528,628
With psychopathic personality	120	1,209,993	50	604,997
With mental deficiency	105	1,082,723	10	108,272
Undiagnosed psychoses	84	836,610	60	501,966
Without psychosis	65	600,088	40	240,035
Total	4,364	$33,293,605		$20,455,673

We have previously seen that the cost of maintenance of hospital cases of mental disease in New York State in 1931 was $44,913,504. Adding this amount to the present worth of the net loss of earnings of the new cases entering the hospitals, we have a grand total of $129,338,773. This amount, if our assumptions are correct, represents the loss in 1931 due to hospital cases of mental disease in New York State.

Economic Loss Due to Mental Disease in the United States

We have still to consider the economic loss on account of mental disease in the United States as a whole. Unfortunately, data are lacking for the complete determination of such loss, and we are compelled to make estimates based on data derived from incomplete censuses and from the results already obtained for New York State.

We estimate the total resident patient population in the hospitals for mental disease in the United States on January 1, 1931, to be 333,317, and the first admissions to such hospitals for the year ended June 30, 1931, to be 97,537, of which 57,432 are estimated to be males and 40,105 females.

For New York State, we found the general average annual per capita cost of maintenance of patients, including hospital care and treatment, housing, and general administration, to be $831.62. In view of the fact that Federal data concerning costs of hospital care and treatment in the United States show that the general average annual per capita cost in all State hospitals is about three-fourths of the cost in New York State hospitals, we have decided to estimate the total annual per capita cost in the United States as three-fourths of that in New York State, or $623.72. On this basis the cost of maintenance of the 333,317 patients in institutions for mental disease in the United States during the year ended June 30, 1931, would be $207,896,479.

Likewise we estimate the loss of future net earnings of the average first admission to hospitals for mental disease in the United States to be three-fourths of the amount found for the average first admission in New York State. We believe such estimate is justifiable, as it is well known that the cost of living and salary and wage scales in New York State are considerably higher than those prevailing in most other states. Referring to Tables 3 and 4, we find the average loss of earnings per first admission in such State to be $9,945.80 for the males and $4,687.37 for the females. Three-fourths of these amounts would be $7,459.35, and $3,515.53, respectively. On this basis the loss of earnings for the 57,432 male first admissions would be $428,405,389 and for the 38,353 female first admissions, $140,990,331. These amounts added to the cost of maintenance as given above make a grand total of $777,292,199. This amount, we believe, constitutes a fair estimate of the economic loss due to hospital cases of mental disease in the United States in the year ended June 30, 1931.

CHAPTER V

The Depression and Mental Disease in New York State*

In October, 1929, occurred a stock market crash of unprecedented magnitude. This economic shock was followed by one of the most severe crises that this country has ever experienced. Millions of men were thrown out of work. Great and small fortunes faded away. Factories, banks and mercantile establishments failed in great numbers. Privation, humiliation, distress and misery came to thousands of homes.

These tremendous changes in economic and social status and in outlook and attitude were accompanied by corresponding emotional stresses. Hope gave way to despair and joy to anxiety. The feeling of security that had grown strong in the days of plenty was lost and was succeeded by apprehension and distrust of the future. Grief over losses of fortunes or positions, fear of poverty and social degradation, and forebodings of evil days to come where accompanied by most distressing mental conflicts.

As the depression has continued in more or less severity for nearly five years, it would naturally have an unfavorable effect on mental health and its results should be reflected in mental hospital statistics.

As uniform statistical data have been compiled for many years by the New York State hospital system it was felt that an analysis of results in such system during the past 10 years might throw some light on the extent to which the depression has been a factor in increasing mental disease.

The census of resident patients in the several classes of hospitals for mental disease in New York State at the end of each of the past 11 years is shown in Table 1. Roughly speaking the years from 1924 to 1929 may be considered as years of prosperity and those from 1929 to 1934 as years of depression. In the first period the total increase of patients was 8,000, or 1,600 per year. In the second period, the total increase was 12,502, or 2,500 per year. The average annual increase in the civil State hospitals in the first period was 1,272 and in the second period 2,411; in the hospitals for criminal insane in the first period, 56, and in the second period, 64;

*Published in American Journal of Psychiatry, January, 1935.

in the licensed institutions, which include two veterans' hospitals, in the first period, 272, and in the second period, 25. Excluding the veterans' hospitals the private licensed institutions had an average increase during the first period of 32 and during the second period of 23.

TABLE 1. RESIDENT PATIENTS IN HOSPITALS FOR MENTAL DISEASE IN NEW YORK STATE AT END OF FISCAL YEAR, 1924-1933

Date June 30	All hospitals	Civil state hospitals	Hospitals for criminal insane	Licensed institutions*
1924	42,469	38,958	1,526	1,985
1925	43,861	40,281	1,556	2,024
1926	45,054	41,337	1,576	2,141
1927	46,802	42,823	1,639	2,340
1928	49,023	44,472	1,752	2,799
1929	50,469	45,319	1,807	3,343
1930	52,612	47,330	1,861	3,421
1931	53,634	48,390	1,937	3,307
1932	57,156	52,364	2,014	2,778
1933	60,493	55,278	2,041	3,174
1934	62,971	57,374	2,128	3,469

*Includes committed and voluntary patients.

Table 2 shows increases in each group of hospitals year by year during the period under consideration. The figures are rather surprising as they show marked augmentation of hospital population during the so-called boom years of 1927 and 1928; in fact, the in-

TABLE 2. INCREASE IN RESIDENT PATIENTS IN HOSPITALS FOR MENTAL DISEASE IN NEW YORK STATE, 1924-1933

Fiscal year ended June 30	All hospitals	Civil state hospitals	Hospitals for criminal insane	Licensed institutions*
1924	1,174	950	19	205
1925	1,418	1,349	30	39
1926	955	818	20	117
1927	2,153	1,891	63	199
1928	2,794	2,222	113	459
1929	2,223	1,624	55	544
1930	2,006	1,874	54	78
1931	1,846	1,884	76	—114
1932	2,438	2,890	77	—529
1933	3,367	2,944	27	396
1934	2,478	2,096	87	295

*Includes committed and voluntary patients.

creases of these two years were greater than those of 1930 and 1931. The opening of new hospitals in 1927 and 1928 may have been a factor in stimulating admissions, but no patients were refused admission in previous years. The increases in the civil state hospitals in 1932 and 1933 broke all records.

Table 3 shows the first admissions to the several groups of hospitals from 1924 to 1933.

TABLE 3. FIRST ADMISSIONS TO HOSPITALS FOR MENTAL DISEASE IN NEW YORK STATE, 1924-1933

Fiscal year ended June 30	All hospitals		Civil state hospitals	Hospitals for criminal insane	Licensed institutions*
	No.	Rate per 100,000 population			
1924	7,435	67.8	6,933	158	344
1925	7,903	71.2	7,435	149	319
1926	7,802	68.8	7,295	133	374
1927	8,554	73.6	7,928	185	441
1928	9,220	77.3	8,614	224	382
1929	9,291	76.0	8,550	182	559
1930	9,581	76.6	9,040	189	352
1931	9,848	76.9	9,286	191	371
1932	10,641	81.2	10,142	202	297
1933	11,354	84.7	10,935	181	238

*Includes committed cases only.

It is generally recognized that the annual rates of first admissions per 100,000 of the general population constitute the best index of the increase of mental disease. Such rates in Table 3 show an irregular upward trend for the period covered. Marked increases in the rate occurred in the years 1925, 1927, 1928, 1932 and 1933. It is noteworthy that the rate was lower in 1930 and in 1931 than in 1928.

Table 4 gives the record with respect to admissions, discharges and deaths. It will be noted that in the nine years the annual admissions increased from 12,035 to 16,167, or 4,135; the annual discharges from 6,854 to 8,019, or 1,165; and the annual deaths from 3,767 to 4,848, or 1,081. The percentages of increase were 34.4, 17.0 and 28.7, respectively. Such a difference in trend between incoming and outgoing cases would naturally lead to marked increases in hospital population. The low rate of increase of discharges during some of the depression years is probably due to the difficulties experienced by the hospitals in finding suitable places for patients ready to be placed on parole.

A clearer understanding of increases in first admissions may be obtained from the consideration of the trends in the principal psychotic groups.

TABLE 4. ADMISSIONS, DISCHARGES AND DEATHS, HOSPITALS FOR MENTAL DISEASE IN NEW YORK STATE, 1924-1933

Fiscal year ended June 30	All admissions, excluding transfers	Discharges	Deaths
1924	12,032	6,854	3,767
1925	12,451	7,037	3,945
1926	12,343	6,997	4,344
1927	12,924	6,695	4,047
1928	13,937	6,983	4,121
1929	14,116	7,361	4,500
1930	14,369	7,847	4,472
1931	14,476	8,113	4,504
1932	15,522	8,349	4,720
1933	16,167	8,019	4,848

Table 5, which gives the record of the senile first admissions from 1924 to 1933, shows only a slight upward trend in absolute numbers and in rate per 100,000 of population. It will be noted, however, that the senile group in 1933 did not constitute as large

TABLE 5. FIRST ADMISSIONS WITH SENILE PSYCHOSES, NEW YORK CIVIL STATE HOSPITALS, 1924-1933

Year	Number			Per cent of first admissions			Number per 100,000 of general population		
	Males	Females	Total	Males	Females	Total	Males	Females	Total
1924	256	421	677	7.0	13.0	9.8	4.7	7.7	6.2
1925	313	443	756	8.1	12.4	10.2	5.7	8.0	6.8
1926	336	420	756	8.5	12.6	10.4	5.9	7.4	6.7
1927	334	439	773	7.7	12.3	9.8	5.7	7.6	6.6
1928	389	513	902	8.2	13.2	10.4	6.5	8.6	7.6
1929	372	470	842	7.9	12.3	9.8	6.1	7.7	6.9
1930	302	494	796	6.1	12.1	8.8	4.8	7.9	6.4
1931	317	435	752	6.2	10.4	8.1	4.9	6.8	5.9
1932	366	517	883	6.5	11.4	8.7	5.6	7.9	6.7
1933	393	550	943	6.5	11.2	8.6	5.8	8.2	7.0

a percentage of all admissions as in 1924. It is probable that certain types of cases formerly diagnosed as senile are now placed in the arteriosclerotic group.

Remarkable changes in the arteriosclerotic group are shown in Table 6. The annual number of first admissions increased from 675 in 1924 to 1,834 in 1933, and the rate per 100,000 from 6.2 to 13.7. The largest increase of any single year occurred in 1932. Part of the increase in this group is undoubtedly due to the advancing age of the general population.

TABLE 6. FIRST ADMISSIONS WITH CEREBRAL ARTERIOSCLEROSIS, NEW YORK CIVIL STATE HOSPITALS, 1924-1933

Year	Number			Per cent of first admissions			Number per 100,000 of general population		
	Males	Females	Total	Males	Females	Total	Males	Females	Total
1924 ...	386	289	675	10.5	8.9	9.7	7.1	5.3	6.2
1925 ...	407	330	737	10.5	9.2	9.9	7.4	5.9	6.6
1926 ...	494	372	866	12.5	11.2	11.9	8.7	6.6	7.6
1927 ...	576	402	978	13.2	11.3	12.3	9.9	6.9	8.4
1928 ...	597	423	1,020	12.6	10.9	11.8	10.0	7.1	8.6
1929 ...	637	493	1,130	13.5	12.9	13.2	10.4	8.1	9.2
1930 ...	746	544	1,290	15.1	13.3	14.3	11.9	8.7	10.3
1931 ...	781	595	1,376	15.3	14.2	14.8	12.2	9.3	10.7
1932 ...	964	720	1,684	17.2	15.8	16.6	14.7	11.0	12.9
1933 ...	1,065	769	1,834	17.7	15.6	16.8	15.8	11.5	13.7

TABLE 7. FIRST ADMISSIONS WITH GENERAL PARALYSIS, NEW YORK CIVIL STATE HOSPITALS, 1924-1933

Year	Number			Per cent of first admissions			Number per 100,000 of general population		
	Males	Females	Total	Males	Females	Total	Males	Females	Total
1924 ...	664	158	822	18.0	4.9	11.9	12.2	2.9	7.5
1925 ...	647	164	811	16.7	4.6	10.9	11.7	2.9	7.3
1926 ...	658	153	811	16.6	4.6	11.1	11.7	2.7	7.2
1927 ...	652	170	822	14.9	4.8	10.4	11.3	2.9	7.1
1928 ...	734	192	926	15.5	4.9	10.7	12.4	3.2	7.8
1929 ...	688	172	860	14.6	4.5	10.1	11.3	2.8	7.0
1930 ...	740	192	932	14.9	4.7	10.3	11.9	3.1	7.4
1931 ...	713	214	927	14.0	5.1	10.0	11.1	3.4	7.2
1932 ...	741	181	922	13.3	4.0	9.1	11.3	2.8	7.0
1933 ...	791	228	1,019	13.2	4.6	9.3	11.8	3.4	7.6

Trends in the general paralysis group are shown in Table 7. First admissions of this psychosis are increasing at a rate approximately the same as that of the general population. Apparently the trend has not been seriously affected by the depression.

Data for the alcoholic group appear in Table 8. A slightly upward trend is found although the changes during the depression period have not been marked. This group is probably more affected by liquor legislation than by economic conditions.

TABLE 8. FIRST ADMISSIONS WITH ALCOHOLIC PSYCHOSES, NEW YORK CIVIL STATE HOSPITALS, 1924-1933

Year	Number			Per cent of first admissions			Number per 100,000 of general population		
	Males	Females	Total	Males	Females	Total	Males	Females	Total
1924 ...	302	71	373	8.2	2.2	5.4	5.5	1.3	3.4
1925 ...	341	81	422	8.8	2.3	5.7	6.2	1.5	3.8
1926 ...	333	89	422	8.4	2.7	5.8	5.9	1.6	3.7
1927 ...	440	114	554	10.1	3.2	7.0	7.6	2.0	4.8
1928 ...	430	79	509	9.1	2.0	5.9	7.2	1.3	4.3
1929 ...	459	78	537	9.7	2.0	6.3	7.5	1.3	4.4
1930 ...	446	100	546	9.0	2.4	6.0	7.1	1.6	4.4
1931 ...	497	102	599	9.8	2.4	6.5	7.7	1.6	4.7
1932 ...	462	131	593	8.3	2.9	5.8	7.0	2.0	4.5
1933 ...	556	150	706	9.3	3.0	6.5	8.3	2.2	5.3

Table 9 deals with the manic-depressive group. The figures reveal only a slight upward trend in rate of first admissions per 100,000 of population. An exceptional increase occurred in 1933.

TABLE 9. FIRST ADMISSIONS WITH MANIC-DEPRESSIVE PSYCHOSES, NEW YORK CIVIL STATE HOSPITALS, 1924-1933

Year	Number			Per cent of first admissions			Number per 100,000 of general population		
	Males	Females	Total	Males	Females	Total	Males	Females	Total
1924 ...	383	619	1,002	10.4	19.0	14.5	7.0	11.3	9.1
1925 ...	359	691	1,050	9.3	19.4	14.1	6.5	12.4	9.5
1926 ...	388	607	995	9.8	18.2	13.6	6.8	10.7	8.8
1927 ...	392	678	1,070	9.0	19.0	13.5	6.7	11.7	9.2
1928 ...	441	755	1,196	9.3	19.4	13.9	7.4	12.7	10.0
1929 ...	437	765	1,202	9.2	20.0	14.1	7.1	12.5	9.8
1930 ...	453	707	1,160	9.1	17.3	12.8	7.2	11.3	9.3
1931 ...	498	707	1,205	9.8	16.9	13.0	7.7	11.1	9.4
1932 ...	489	742	1,231	8.7	16.3	12.1	7.4	11.4	9.4
1933 ...	548	862	1,410	9.1	17.5	12.9	8.1	12.9	10.5

Ever since 1927 a distinct rise in trend in the dementia præcox group has been noted. The most significant change occurred in 1932. The high rate of first admissions of that year, however, was exceeded by that of 1933.

TABLE 10. FIRST ADMISSIONS WITH DEMENTIA PRÆCOX, NEW YORK CIVIL STATE HOSPITALS, 1924-1933

Year	Number			Per cent of first admissions			Number per 100,000 of general population		
	Males	Females	Total	Males	Females	Total	Males	Females	Total
1924 ...	1,003	910	1,913	27.2	28.0	27.6	18.4	16.6	17.5
1925 ...	1,068	990	2,058	27.6	27.7	27.7	19.3	17.8	18.5
1926 ...	1,045	901	1,946	26.3	27.1	26.7	18.5	15.8	17.2
1927 ...	1,197	952	2,149	27.4	26.7	27.1	20.7	16.3	18.5
1928 ...	1,261	1,065	2,326	26.7	27.4	27.0	21.2	17.8	19.5
1929 ...	1,174	988	2,162	24.8	25.8	25.3	19.3	16.1	17.7
1930 ...	1,299	1,070	2,369	26.2	26.2	26.2	20.8	17.0	18.9
1931 ...	1,302	1,140	2,442	25.5	27.2	26.3	20.3	17.9	19.1
1932 ...	1,486	1,269	2,755	26.6	27.9	27.2	22.6	19.4	21.0
1933 ...	1,482	1,360	2,842	24.7	27.6	26.0	22.0	20.4	21.2

Judging from the data concerning the six principal groups presented in Tables 5-10, the economic crisis does not appear to be the dominant factor in the increase of first admissions to our State hospitals. That it has been a precipitating factor of significance no one can doubt. Definite evidence of the fact is furnished by reports of etiological factors appearing in the history of first admissions from 1924 to 1933.

Cases in which loss of position or financial loss was clearly an etiological factor are shown in Table 11 for each year of the period studied. As would be expected such cases were more numerous during the depression years, a decidedly upward trend being noted from 1929 to 1933. In the last year the cases comprised 8.8 per cent of all admissions as compared with 2.2 per cent in 1924.

The data in Table 11, of course, cannot be construed as indicating the entire effect of the depression on admissions. Many of the influences of the depression are too indefinite to be counted as causal factors, but, nevertheless, are not without significance.

TABLE 11. CASES AMONG FIRST ADMISSIONS IN WHICH LOSS OF POSITION OR FINANCIAL LOSS WAS REPORTED AS AN ETIOLOGICAL FACTOR, NEW YORK CIVIL STATE HOSPITALS

Year	Number	Per cent
1924	151	2.2
1925	151	2.0
1926	183	2.5
1927	145	1.8
1928	157	1.8
1929	209	2.4
1930	281	3.1
1931	438	4.7
1932	639	6.3
1933	958	8.8

CONCLUSIONS

1. Patient population of mental hospitals in New York State increased more rapidly from 1929 to 1934 than from 1924 to 1929. The increase was greatest in 1933.

2. The trend in the rate of first admissions has been rising since 1924.

3. The rate of increase of admissions is higher than that of discharges and deaths.

4. A slight upward trend is noted in senile first admissions.

5. Extraordinary increases have occurred in the arteriosclerotic group during the past 10 years. The most marked change was in 1932.

6. No change in trend is found in the paretic group.

7. A slowly rising trend is noted in the alcoholic group. The group is more affected by liquor legislation than by economic conditions.

8. The trend in the manic-depressive first admissions is slightly upward. A marked increase occurred in this group in 1933.

9. A significant increase in the rate of dementia præcox first admissions has occurred since 1927. The rate was exceptionally high in 1932 and 1933. Such rate may reflect cumulative effects of the depression.

10. The economic crisis does not seem to be the dominant factor in the increase of first admissions in any one diagnostic group; it is, however, a precipitating factor of importance in all groups.

CHAPTER VI

Trends in Outcome of General Paresis*

During 1925 to 1931 the treatment of general paresis in New York civil State hospitals underwent a remarkable transformation. Through the efficacy of the newer methods of treatment, a fatal disease became curable and hope displaced despair in the minds of many afflicted persons. In this wonderful achievement, modern medical science adds another victory to its long list of triumphs over disease and death.

Many scientific papers have been published showing results in the treatment of groups of patients by tryparsamide, malaria, radiothermy and diathermy. Such communications, valuable as they are, give a detailed view of only part of the picture. To comprehend fully the results of the newer methods of treatment, it is also necessary to have a general view of outcome with respect to all cases.

With this thought in mind we have studied the statistical history of the first admissions to our civil State hospitals for the years 1920 to 1931, inclusive. We stopped with 1931 as we desired to have a four-year period of observation for all cases. As the newer methods of treatment were adopted to a considerable extent in 1925, the fiscal years, 1920-1925 may be taken as the period ''before treatment'' and the years 1926-1931 as the period ''after treatment''. The difference in results in the two periods is truly remarkable.

Other bases of comparison are found in studies of outcome in general paralysis cases made by Dr. Mortimer W. Raynor and by Raymond G. Fuller. In June, 1923, Dr. Raynor presented at an interhospital conference held at Manhattan State Hospital a paper entitled ''Remissions in General Paralysis''. The paper was based on a study of 1,004 male first admissions with general paralysis received at the Manhattan State Hospital during the period from July 1, 1911 to June 30, 1918. These patients were considered by Dr. Raynor as untreated cases as they had received no special treatment by use of arsenical preparations. Of the 1,004 patients, 882, or 87.8 per cent, had died previous to the date of the study;

*Read at Quarterly Conference of New York State Department of Mental Hygiene at Albany, March 23, 1935.

40 cases were known to be living; the status of 20 that had been discharged was unknown and 62 cases had been deported; 33, or 3.5 per cent, of the cases had had remissions. Of these, 19 had later died; 85 patients, or 9.0 per cent of the total, had left the hospital as improved.

The study by Mr. Fuller was entitled "Expectation of Hospital Life and Outcome of Mental Patients on First Admission" and was published in the Psychiatric Quarterly for April, 1930. This study dealt with general paralysis as well as other principal psychoses. The data with respect to general paralysis were obtained by studying the statistical history of 600 male and 600 female paretic first admissions to the New York civil State hospitals received during a period directly following October 1, 1909. As these cases were admitted before the introduction of salvarsan, they could all be considered untreated cases. Mr. Fuller found that 75.5 per cent of the male patients with general paralysis had died in the hospitals within four years and 81.3 per cent within 15 years. Of the female cases, 59.8 per cent had died within four years and 67.2 per cent within 15 years; 14.3 per cent of the males and 21.0 per cent of the females had been discharged within 15 years.

According to Mr. Fuller's findings at the end of 15 years, 8.1 per cent of the patients with general paralysis remained in the hospitals; 74.3 per cent had died in the hospitals and 17.7 per cent had been discharged and had not returned.

The figures compiled by both Dr. Raynor and Mr. Fuller indicate clearly the generally hopeless prognosis of general paresis that had prevailed for many years prior to 1925.

The present study comprises 10,240 first admissions, of whom 8,186 were males and 2,054 females. (See Table 1.) There has been a slight upward trend in the annual *number* of first admissions during the years studied but the *rate* per 100,000 of population decreased from 7.9 in 1920 to 7.2 in 1931. Among the females, however, the rate increased from 2.7 in 1920 to 3.4 in 1931. The upward trend in discharges and the downward trend in deaths are clearly evident in the data set forth in the table. These will be more fully shown in later tables.

Attention is called to the fact that 1,439 patients, first admitted during the 12-year period under consideration, were still in the hos-

TABLE 1. OUTCOME OF FIRST ADMISSIONS WITH GENERAL PARESIS, 1920-1931

Year	Total first admissions			Discharges			Readmissions			Deaths			Remaining in hospital, February 1, 1935		
	Males	Females	Total	Males	Females	Total	Males	Females	Total	Males	Females	Total	Males	Females	Total
1920	683	142	825	105	31	136	42	10	52	599	110	709	13	8	21
1921	671	159	830	111	36	147	37	8	45	578	123	701	18	5	23
1922	661	174	835	111	35	146	27	20	47	541	138	679	31	17	48
1923	655	144	799	107	34	141	37	17	54	550	119	669	30	11	41
1924	664	161	825	126	39	165	31	10	41	516	105	621	49	25	74
1925	658	170	828	146	47	193	13	12	25	471	110	581	58	23	81
1926	656	154	810	186	54	240	37	12	49	407	86	493	90	23	113
1927	645	175	820	221	46	267	32	4	36	353	100	453	93	32	125
1928	736	193	929	236	73	309	30	12	42	363	87	450	171	41	212
1929	692	177	869	216	64	280	24	9	33	356	87	443	139	33	172
1930	743	193	936	236	77	313	26	17	43	326	74	400	205	57	262
1931	722	212	934	238	75	313	27	9	36	297	87	384	212	55	267
Total ..	8,186	2,054	10,240	2,039	611	2,650	363	140	503	5,357	1,226	6,583	1,109	330	1,439

pitals on February 1, 1935. These cases comprised 13.5 per cent of the males, and 16.1 per cent of the females.

Age Distribution

To show possible trends in ages of first admissions during the period, we have computed the per cent distribution by age groups and sex for each year. The results appear in Table 2. Considerable variation from year to year is found in both sexes. This

Table 2. Per Cent Distribution by Age Groups of First Admissions with General Paresis, 1920-1931

Year	Total first admissions	Age groups							
		Under 20 years	20-29 years	30-39 years	40-49 years	50-59 years	60-69 years	70 years and over	Unascertained
				Males					
1920 ...	683	0.6	3.5	34.7	34.1	21.5	5.6	...	...
1921 ...	671	0.1	4.5	34.0	38.2	17.4	5.2	0.6	...
1922 ...	661	0.5	4.1	32.2	37.1	18.5	7.0	0.6	0.2
1923 ...	655	...	5.0	31.5	37.1	20.9	5.0	0.5	...
1924 ...	664	0.2	4.2	33.1	33.1	22.0	6.6	0.6	0.2
1925 ...	658	0.5	4.4	30.7	36.8	20.5	6.4	0.8	...
1926 ...	656	0.3	3.5	34.1	36.0	18.9	5.5	1.2	0.5
1927 ...	645	0.3	4.3	27.9	40.2	20.5	6.4	0.3	0.2
1928 ...	736	0.3	4.8	30.7	37.4	20.1	6.0	0.8	...
1929 ...	692	0.6	3.2	28.9	36.4	21.7	8.1	1.2	...
1930 ...	743	0.4	4.6	30.8	36.7	20.2	6.3	0.9	...
1931 ...	722	0.7	5.4	27.7	36.8	21.6	6.5	1.1	0.1
Total..	8,186	0.4	4.3	31.3	36.6	20.3	6.2	0.7	0.1
				Females					
1920 ...	142	0.7	9.9	28.2	32.4	25.4	3.5	...	...
1921 ...	159	1.9	9.4	32.7	34.0	17.0	5.0	...	...
1922 ...	174	0.6	11.5	35.1	28.2	18.4	5.2	1.1	...
1923 ...	144	0.7	12.5	29.2	37.5	14.6	5.6	...	...
1924 ...	161	0.6	8.7	30.4	37.3	18.0	4.3	0.6	...
1925 ...	170	1.8	5.9	30.6	34.1	20.6	7.1	...	...
1926 ...	154	0.6	7.1	23.4	35.7	25.3	5.8	1.9	...
1927 ...	175	2.3	10.3	27.4	36.0	16.6	6.3	1.1	...
1928 ...	193	3.1	8.8	24.4	38.3	17.1	6.2	1.6	0.5
1929 ...	177	0.6	9.0	24.9	39.0	16.9	9.0	0.6	...
1930 ...	193	2.6	11.4	31.6	29.5	19.2	4.1	1.6	...
1931 ...	212	2.4	6.6	34.9	32.5	16.5	6.1	0.9	...
Total..	2,054	1.6	9.2	29.5	34.5	18.6	5.7	0.8	*

*Less than 0.05 per cent.

would be expected as the numbers in the several age groups are not large. It will be noted that in the groups under 30 years of age, the percentages of females are much larger than those of the males. Of the whole number studied, 88.2 per cent of the males and 82.6 per cent of the females were between 30 and 60 years of age at time of first admission. About two-thirds of the patients are admitted during the fourth and fifth decades of life. No marked trends in age distribution are observable in the period studied.

TABLE 3. DURATION OF HOSPITAL LIFE PREVIOUS TO FIRST DISCHARGE OF FIRST ADMISSIONS WITH GENERAL PARESIS, 1920-1931

Year	Total first admissions	Total dis-charges	Duration of hospital life				
			Under 6 months	6-11 months	12-17 months	18-23 months	24 months and over
			Males				
1920	683	105	67	21	7	5	5
1921	671	111	77	12	6	5	11
1922	661	111	70	17	11	5	8
1923	655	107	67	23	8	2	7
1924	661	126	67	28	14	8	9
1925	658	146	74	31	14	9	18
1926	656	186	83	46	26	14	17
1927	645	221	95	57	30	17	22
1928	736	236	99	67	32	10	28
1929	692	216	111	64	27	4	10
1930	743	236	133	63	18	8	14
1931	722	238	133	66	19	10	10
Total..	8,186	2,039	1,076	495	212	97	159
			Females				
1920	142	31	19	9	..	..	3
1921	159	36	19	8	5	3	1
1922	174	35	21	9	3	1	1
1923	144	34	21	5	3	3	2
1924	161	39	10	13	6	2	8
1925	170	47	19	16	4	2	6
1926	154	54	26	12	11	1	4
1927	175	46	13	20	6	1	6
1928	193	73	37	16	7	7	6
1929	177	64	39	11	10	..	4
1930	193	77	46	17	9	3	2
1931	212	75	42	24	4	2	3
Total..	2,054	611	312	160	68	25	46

Discharges

Table 3 classifies discharges of each year by duration of hospital life. Of the males, 24.9 per cent, and of the females 29.7 per cent, were discharged during the period elapsing from time of admission to February 1, 1935. More than half of the discharges occurred within 6 months following admission. The upward trend of discharges during the period studied is clearly evident among both males and females. Correspondingly, there is a trend toward shorter duration of hospital life.

Table 4. Condition on First Discharge of First Admissions with General Paresis, 1920-1931

Year	Total first admissions	Total discharges	Condition on discharge				
			Recovered	Much Improved	Improved	Unimproved	Others
			Males				
1920	683	105	3	28	37	37	..
1921	671	111	1	32	33	45	..
1922	661	111	3	37	37	34	..
1923	655	107	1	37	41	28	..
1924	664	126	2	50	31	43	..
1925	658	146	2	70	42	32	..
1926	656	186	7	96	54	27	2
1927	645	221	12	86	75	48	..
1928	736	236	5	123	80	27	1
1929	692	216	3	112	75	26	..
1930	743	236	11	134	71	20	..
1931	722	238	20	96	93	29	..
Total..	8,186	2,039	70	901	669	396	3
			Females				
1920	142	31	..	9	13	9	..
1921	159	36	..	13	11	12	..
1922	174	35	2	12	11	10	..
1923	144	34	..	13	13	6	2
1924	161	39	4	20	10	5	..
1925	170	47	3	21	10	13	..
1926	154	54	5	21	23	5	..
1927	175	46	6	15	20	5	..
1928	193	73	4	32	27	10	..
1929	177	64	3	30	25	6	..
1930	193	77	6	37	28	5	1
1931	212	75	2	40	24	9	..
Total..	2,054	611	35	263	215	95	3

A more significant story is told by Table 4. Here is given a definite accounting of the beneficent effects of the newer methods of treatment. Comparing results among males of 1920 with those of 1931, we note 3 recoveries among the cases of the former year and 20 among those of the latter; 28 much improved cases of the former year, and 96 of the latter; 37 improved cases of the former year, and 93 of the latter. Similar contrasts are seen in the figures relating to females.

TRENDS IN IMPROVEMENT AND DEATH RATES PER 100 OF MALE FIRST ADMISSIONS, 1920-1931

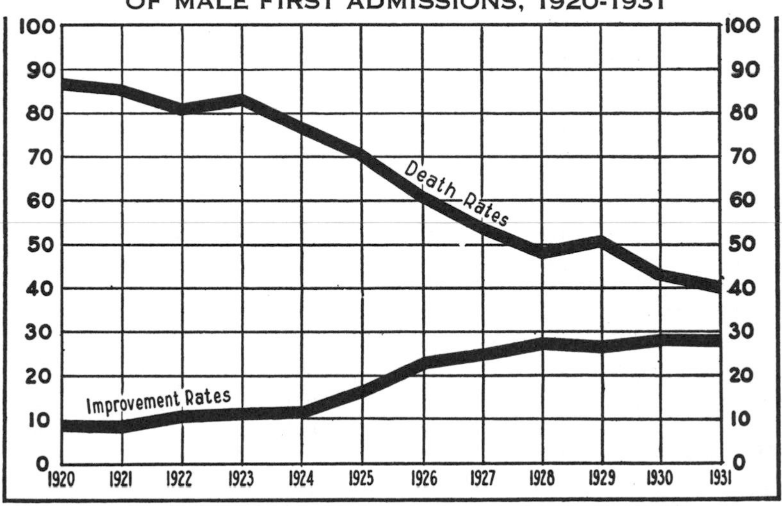

Chart 1.

In Table 5, rates of recovery and improvement per 100 first admissions are given for each year from 1920 to 1931. The rates under each heading vary but little from 1920 to 1924. Gains in improvement are noted in 1925 and more marked gains in the succeeding years. The table relating to males shows that of the 1920 first admissions, only 9.9 per cent were discharged as benefited by treatment. Of the 1930 admissions 29.1 per cent were so discharged. Had the former rates prevailed with respect to the 1931 admissions the number of male first admissions of that year who were later discharged benefited by treatment would have been 71 instead of 209.

TABLE 5. RATES OF RECOVERY AND IMPROVEMENT PER 100 OF FIRST ADMISSIONS WITH GENERAL PARESIS, 1920-1931

Year	Total first admissions	Condition on discharge*			
		Recovered	Much improved	Improved	Unimproved
		Males			
1920	683	0.4	4.1	5.4	5.4
1921	671	0.1	4.8	4.9	6.7
1922	661	0.5	5.6	5.6	5.1
1923	655	0.2	5.6	6.3	4.3
1924	664	0.3	7.5	4.7	6.5
1925	658	0.3	10.6	6.4	4.9
1926	656	1.1	14.6	8.2	4.1
1927	645	1.9	13.3	11.6	7.4
1928	736	0.7	16.7	10.9	3.7
1929	692	0.4	16.2	10.8	3.8
1930	743	1.5	18.0	9.6	2.7
1931	722	2.8	13.3	12.9	4.0
Total	8,186	0.9	11.0	8.2	4.8
		Females			
1920	142	..	6.3	9.2	6.3
1921	159	..	8.2	6.9	7.5
1922	174	1.1	6.9	6.3	5.7
1923	144	..	9.0	9.0	4.2
1924	161	2.5	12.4	6.2	3.1
1925	170	1.8	12.4	5.9	7.6
1926	154	3.2	13.6	14.9	3.2
1927	175	3.4	8.6	11.4	2.9
1928	193	2.1	16.6	14.0	5.2
1929	177	1.7	16.9	14.1	3.4
1930	193	3.1	19.2	14.5	2.6
1931	212	0.9	18.9	11.3	4.2
Total	2,054	1.7	12.8	10.5	4.6

*In addition 6 cases were otherwise discharged.

Among females in general the rate of patients discharged as benefited by treatment is much higher than that found among males. Of the 1920 female first admissions, 6.3 per cent were discharged as much improved and 9.2 per cent as improved, a total of 15.5 per cent. This is in contrast with 9.9 per cent of the males of the same year. Of the 1930 female first admissions, 36.8 per cent were discharged as benefited by treatment. Considering the serious nature of the disease and the fact that many patients are admitted in a critical condition, the latter results are truly remarkable. The trend in rates of improvement shown by this table is very encouraging.

As age is a factor in promoting improvement and recovery, we have tabulated condition on discharge by age groups. The results are shown in Tables 6 and 7. In both males and females the highest rates of recovery and improvement are shown in the age groups between 20 and 40. The rates decline in the succeeding decades. Gratifying results, however, are obtained with patients in the groups from 40 to 70 years of age.

TABLE 6. CONDITION ON FIRST DISCHARGE OF FIRST ADMISSIONS WITH GENERAL PARESIS, CLASSIFIED BY AGE GROUPS, 1920-1931

Age groups, years	Total first admissions	Total dis-charges	Condition on discharge				
			Recovered	Much improved	Improved	Unimproved	Others
			Males				
Under 20....	30	10	1	3	3	3	..
20-29........	352	127	3	52	46	26	..
30-39........	2,565	785	28	353	246	158	..
40-49........	3,000	738	27	344	231	133	3
50-59........	1,664	315	9	127	121	58	..
60-69........	509	60	2	22	21	15	..
70 and over...	59	3	..	..	1	2	..
Unascertained	7	1	..	..	..	1	..
Total......	8,186	2,039	70	901	669	396	3
			Females				
Under 20....	32	18	..	6	5	7	..
20-29........	189	66	6	25	22	12	1
30-39........	606	208	14	98	66	30	..
40-49........	708	208	9	89	85	24	1
50-59........	383	98	6	38	34	20	..
60-69........	118	13	..	7	3	2	1
70 and over...	17	..	..	..	..	..	..
Unascertained	1	..	..	..	..	..	..
Total......	2,054	611	35	263	215	95	3

TRENDS IN IMPROVEMENT AND DEATH RATES PER 100 OF FEMALE FIRST ADMISSIONS 1920-1931

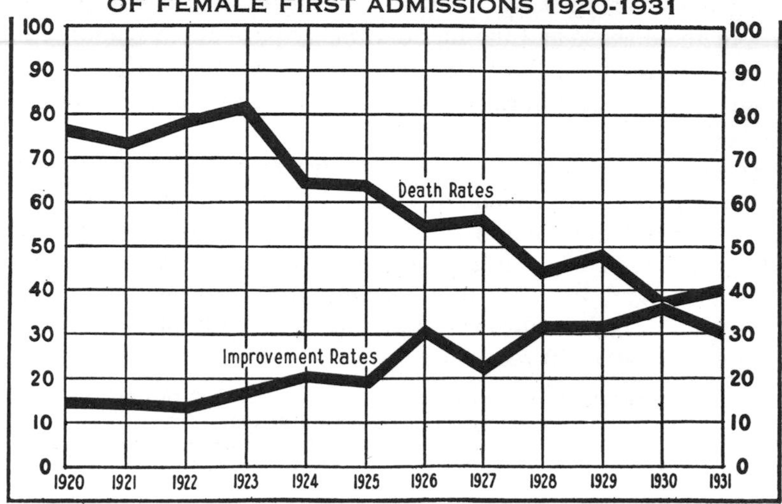

Chart 2.

RATES OF RECOVERY AND IMPROVEMENT PER 100 OF MALE FIRST ADMISSIONS WITH GENERAL PARESIS, 1920 AND 1931

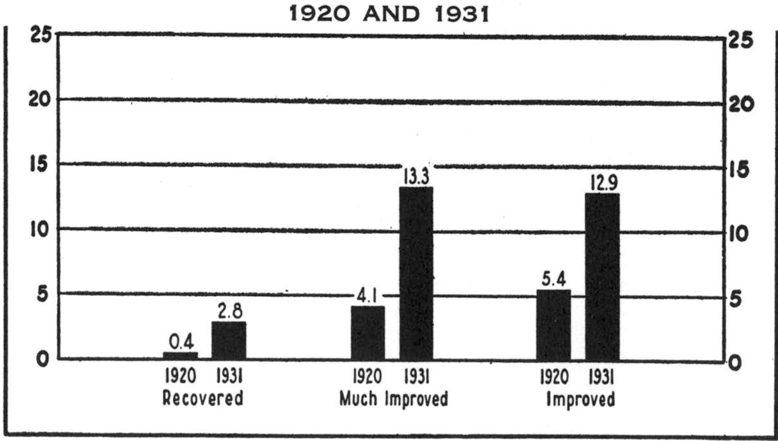

Chart 3.

TABLE 7. RATES OF RECOVERY AND IMPROVEMENT PER 100 OF FIRST ADMISSIONS WITH GENERAL PARESIS, CLASSIFIED BY AGE GROUPS, 1920-1931

Age groups, years	Condition on discharge			
	Recovered	Much improved	Improved	Unimproved
		Males		
20-29	0.9	14.8	13.1	7.4
30-39	1.1	13.8	9.6	6.2
40-49	0.9	11.5	7.7	4.4
50-59	0.5	7.6	7.3	3.5
60-69	0.4	4.3	4.1	2.9
Total discharges	0.9	11.0	8.2	4.8
		Females		
20-29	3.2	13.2	11.6	6.3
30-39	2.3	16.2	10.9	5.0
40-49	1.3	12.6	12.0	3.4
50-59	1.6	9.9	8.9	5.2
60-69	..	5.9	2.5	1.7
Total discharges	1.7	12.8	10.5	4.6

DEATHS

The newer forms of treatment while promoting recovery and improvement naturally lower the death rate. In a study made by the author in 1923, concerning general paresis in New York State, 1913-1922, it was found that the deaths in the hospitals from this disease amounted to 87.7 per cent of the first admissions. In other words the disease proved fatal in the hospitals in an average of 7 out of 8 cases. Dr. Raynor, in the study previously referred to, reported a death rate of 87.8 for the period covered.

Referring to Table 8, we note that 599 of the 683 male first admissions of 1920 died in the hospitals. The rate was the same as that above mentioned namely, 87.7 per cent. The death rate within four years was 82.1 per cent. The death rate among the male first admissions of 1931 for a like period was 41.0 per cent, practically half of that found among the first admissions of 1920.

Of the 683 male first admissions of 1920, 561 died within four years following admission. Of the 722 male first admissions of

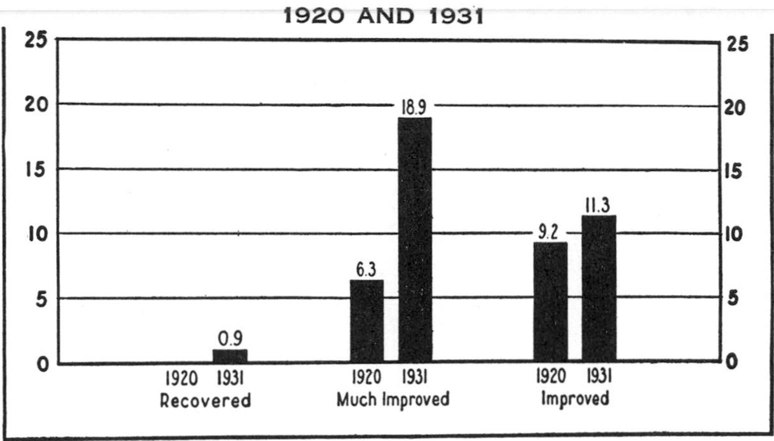

Chart 4.

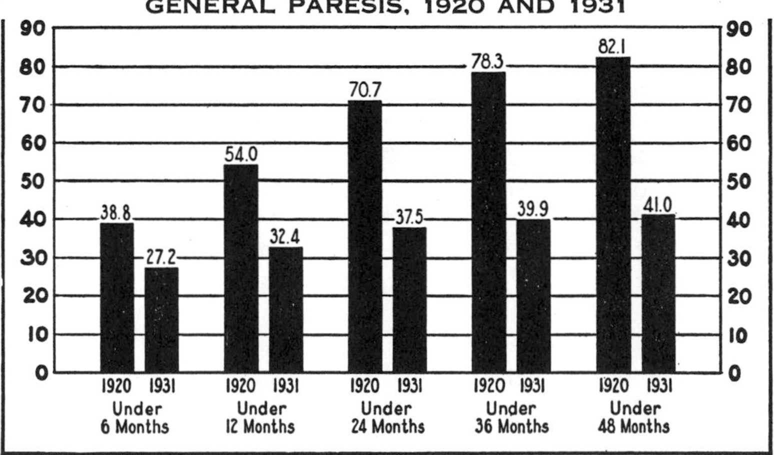

Chart 5.

1931, 296 died within a like period. In the former smaller group the deaths within four years exceeded those of the latter group by 265. A mere glance at Table 8 is sufficient to reveal the great saving in human life that was effected by the newer methods of treatment of general paresis in the State hospitals from 1926 to 1931.

TABLE 8. DEATHS OF FIRST ADMISSIONS WITH GENERAL PARESIS CLASSIFIED BY DURATION OF HOSPITAL LIFE, 1920-1931

Year	Total first admissions	Total deaths	Duration of hospital life						
			Under 6 months	6-11 months	12-17 months	18-23 months	24-35 months	36-47 months	48 months and over
			Males						
1920 ...	683	599	265	104	71	43	52	26	38
1921 ...	671	578	234	104	71	54	58	24	33
1922 ...	661	541	221	88	72	38	61	23	38
1923 ...	655	550	246	93	64	44	57	16	30
1924 ...	664	516	207	80	77	40	51	28	33
1925 ...	658	471	210	84	48	37	36	14	42
1926 ...	656	407	216	60	27	23	29	14	38
1927 ...	645	353	190	56	32	16	18	15	26
1928 ...	736	363	206	41	29	12	28	14	33
1929 ...	692	356	200	52	26	13	25	27	13
1930 ...	743	326	201	46	16	11	22	17	13
1931 ...	722	297	196	38	25	12	17	8	1
Total..	8,186	5,357	2,592	846	558	343	454	226	338
			Females						
1920 ...	142	110	57	9	13	7	9	1	14
1921 ...	159	123	46	17	17	10	16	6	11
1922 ...	174	138	63	21	15	9	10	8	12
1923 ...	144	119	43	19	14	10	17	4	12
1924 ...	161	105	41	13	15	8	11	7	10
1925 ...	170	110	57	12	7	7	14	7	6
1926 ...	154	86	44	15	11	1	3	5	7
1927 ...	175	100	46	13	8	10	8	4	11
1928 ...	193	87	45	12	9	3	2	4	12
1929 ...	177	87	60	6	7	2	5	3	4
1930 ...	193	74	39	12	4	5	4	6	4
1931 ...	212	87	52	12	8	3	7	5	..
Total..	2,054	1,226	593	161	128	75	106	60	103

In order that exact comparisons might be made of death rates during various periods of hospital life, results are set forth on a percentage basis in Table 9. The rates under the various headings in the table are cumulative so that complete rates for 6 months, 12 months, 24 months, 36 months and 48 months are given for the first admissions of each year.

TABLE 9. DEATH RATES PER 100 OF FIRST ADMISSIONS WITH GENERAL PARESIS, CLASSIFIED BY DURATION OF HOSPITAL LIFE, 1920-1931

Year	Death rates by duration of hospital life				
	Under 6 months	Under 12 months	Under 24 months	Under 36 months	Under 48 months
		Males			
1920	38.8	54.0	70.7	78.3	82.1
1921	34.9	50.4	69.0	77.6	81.2
1922	33.4	46.8	63.4	72.6	76.1
1923	37.6	51.8	68.2	77.0	79.4
1924	31.2	43.2	60.8	68.5	72.7
1925	31.9	44.7	57.6	63.1	65.2
1926	32.9	42.1	49.7	54.1	56.3
1927	29.5	38.1	45.6	48.4	50.7
1928	28.0	33.6	39.1	42.9	44.8
1929	28.9	36.4	42.1	45.7	49.6
1930	27.1	33.2	36.9	39.8	42.1
1931	27.2	32.4	37.5	39.9	41.0
Total	31.7	42.0	53.0	58.6	61.3
		Females			
1920	40.1	46.5	60.6	66.9	67.6
1921	28.9	39.6	56.6	66.7	70.4
1922	36.2	48.3	62.1	67.8	72.4
1923	29.9	43.1	59.7	71.5	74.3
1924	25.5	33.5	47.8	54.7	59.0
1925	33.5	40.6	48.8	57.1	61.2
1926	28.6	38.3	46.1	48.1	51.3
1927	26.3	33.7	44.0	48.6	50.9
1928	23.3	29.5	35.8	36.8	38.9
1929	33.9	37.3	42.4	45.2	46.9
1930	20.2	26.4	31.1	33.2	36.3
1931	24.5	30.2	35.4	38.7	41.0
Total	28.9	36.7	46.6	51.8	54.7

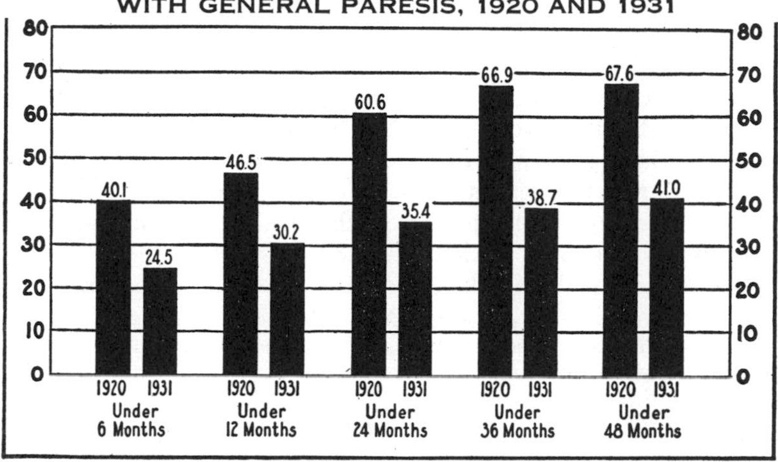

Chart 6.

Of the male first admissions of 1920, 38.8 per cent, died within the first six months of hospital life; 54 per cent within the first year; 70.7 per cent within two years; 78.3 per cent within three years and 82.1 per cent within four years. Of the male first admissions of 1931, 27.2 per cent died within six months; 32.4 per cent within one year; 37.5 per cent within two years, 39.9 per cent within three years and 41 per cent within four years.

Death rates of female first admissions with general paresis average lower than those for male first admissions during the period under consideration. For the last year of the period, however, the rates among males and females were nearly equal. In general a decline in the rates among females has been similar to that among males although the percentage reduction in the rates among females is less. The general trend in death rates among both males and females is downward and we should expect still lower rates for this psychotic group in future years, as treatment becomes standardized and is made available to a larger percentage of cases.

In order to show more definitely the changes in death rates that have occurred during the latter part of the period studied, we have compiled Tables 10 and 11. Table 10 shows death rates for certain age groups classified for various periods of hospital life for the first admissions from 1920 to 1925 inclusive. Table 11 gives similar data for the first admissions of the years from 1926 to 1931 inclusively. The one period comprises roughly the first six years of the newer treatment and the other period the last six years of the older methods of treatment. The contrasts in rates for the two periods are most striking. For the first period the admissions numbered 4,895 and the deaths 3,924. For the second period the admissions numbered 5,199 and the deaths, 2,560. The number of admissions for the first period were 304 less than those for the second period but the number of deaths were 1,364 greater.

TABLE 10. DEATH RATES IN CERTAIN AGE GROUPS PER 100 OF FIRST ADMISSIONS WITH GENERAL PARESIS, CLASSIFIED BY DURATION OF HOSPITAL LIFE, 1920-1925

Age on admission, years	Total first admissions	Total deaths	Duration of hospital life				
			Under 6 months	Under 12 months	Under 24 months	Under 36 months	Under 48 months
			Males				
20-29	171	120	24.0	35.1	49.7	60.8	63.7
30-39	1,306	996	32.2	45.0	60.3	67.5	71.1
40-49	1,439	1,194	34.2	48.0	65.8	74.2	77.1
50-59	804	696	37.6	52.1	69.7	77.6	81.3
60-69	238	220	45.8	65.1	79.0	85.3	88.7
Total ..	3,958	3,226	34.5	48.3	64.9	72.8	76.1
			Females				
20-29	91	58	18.7	30.8	40.7	51.6	53.8
30-39	296	216	28.7	37.2	51.0	60.8	66.2
40-49	321	236	33.3	42.1	58.3	64.2	67.0
50-59	180	146	43.3	52.2	66.7	71.7	75.0
60-69	49	42	38.8	57.1	63.3	77.6	77.6
Total ..	937	698	32.7	42.2	56.1	64.0	67.6

It is noteworthy that for nearly every age group and every period of hospital life, the death rate in the latter period was considerably lower than in the earlier period. Among males in the age group 20-29 years the death rate within 4 years in the first period was 63.7, and in second period 30.9. The corresponding rates among females were 53.8 and 33.7. Similar contrasts in rates are seen for the other age groups. Naturally, the effects of the newer treatment on the death rate become less as the age of the patients advances.

TABLE 11. DEATH RATES IN CERTAIN AGE GROUPS PER 100 OF FIRST ADMISSIONS WITH GENERAL PARESIS, CLASSIFIED BY DURATION OF HOSPITAL LIFE, 1926-1931

Age on admission, years	Total first admissions	Total deaths	Duration of hospital life				
			Under 6 months	Under 12 months	Under 24 months	Under 36 months	Under 48 months
			Males				
20-29	181	62	18.2	22.7	26.0	30.4	30.9
30-39	1,259	512	22.6	27.8	32.6	35.1	36.9
40-49	1,561	753	27.7	34.8	40.7	43.5	45.6
50-59	860	520	34.9	43.0	49.9	54.5	58.1
60-69	271	207	48.7	60.1	66.4	71.6	73.8
Total ..	4,132	2,054	28.6	35.5	41.2	44.5	46.8
			Females				
20-29	98	36	16.3	22.4	28.6	30.6	33.7
30-39	310	106	18.1	22.3	26.1	28.7	31.3
40-49	387	182	27.9	33.3	39.0	41.6	42.6
50-59	203	126	36.0	41.9	49.8	53.2	59.1
60-69	69	56	34.8	53.6	75.4	76.8	76.8
Total ..	1,067	506	26.0	32.1	38.7	41.3	43.9

CONCLUSIONS

1. The trend in rate of male first admissions with general paresis is slowly declining but the trend in female first admissions is rising.

2. No change is found in trend in age distribution of first admissions with general paresis.

3. Trends in recovery and improvement in general paresis cases are upward.

4. Trends in death rates in general paresis cases are downward.

5. Noteworthy gains are found in results of treatment in all age groups of both sexes during the period 1926 to 1931 as compared with the period from 1920 to 1925.

REFERENCES

Fuller, Raymond G.: Expectation of Hospital Life and Outcome for Mental Patients on First Admission. PSYCHIATRIC QUARTERLY, 1930, 4; 295.

Pollock, Horatio M.: General Paralysis in New York State, 1913-1922. STATE HOSPITAL QUARTERLY, 1923, 9; 24.

Raynor, Mortimer W.: Remissions in General Paralysis. STATE HOSPITAL QUARTERLY, 1924, 10; 67.

CHAPTER VII

Recurrence of Attacks in Manic-Depressive Psychoses*

In making statistical studies involving the life cycle of patients the lack of complete data becomes a serious handicap. In the statistical files of the New York State Department of Mental Hygiene there are important facts concerning the hospital life of our patients but nothing at all relative to their life outside of the hospital after discharge, unless, perchance, they return for further treatment.

In studying manic-depressive psychoses, especially, we feel the need of more complete data relative to the patients that recover from the first attack and do not reappear on the hospital records.

The brief study of the recurrence of attacks in manic-depressive psychoses presented herewith was made from the file of statistical cards of the department covering the period from October 1, 1909 to June 30, 1920. The manic-depressive file contains in order of identification number the first admission cards of all patients of this group admitted to the civil State hospitals during such period, together with the subsequent discharge, readmission and death cards relating to the same patients. All cards referring to the same patient are brought together in the file. The cards for the years mentioned give a statistical record of over 8,000 manic-depressive cases.

The purpose of the study is to throw light on the prognosis of manic-depressive psychoses by answering as definitely as possible the following questions:

1. To what extent do recurrent attacks occur in this form of mental disease?
2. To what extent does the recurrence of attacks differ in the several types?
3. How does the recurrence of attacks differ in the various age groups of first admissions?
4. What is the average duration of illness in successive attacks?

A study along somewhat similar lines, made by Dr. Arthur S. Moore of the Middletown (New York) State Hospital, was published in the *State Hospitals Bulletin* in September, 1909. The

*Read at the eighty-seventh annual meeting of The American Psychiatric Association, held in Toronto, Canada, June 2 to 5, 1931.

basis of this study was 100 manic-depressive cases admitted to the Middletown State Hospital during the six years ended January 1, 1909. Another study of prognosis in manic-depressive psychoses made by Dr. J. B. Macdonald of the Danvers (Mass.) State Hospital in 1915, was published in the *Journal of Nervous and Mental Disease* in January, 1918. This study dealt with 451 consecutive first admissions to the Danvers State Hospital.

A wide disparity in results is found in these two studies and neither study agrees very closely with the results obtained from our tabulations. Some of the most striking differences will be referred to in the course of the discussion.

Question 1.—*To what extent do recurrent attacks occur in manic-depressive psychoses?*

To answer this question as completely as possible from the data at hand we tabulated the number of attacks reported at time of last admission for the admissions of 11 fiscal years.

The cases were classified according to type at last admission, and the cases unascertained with respect to type and number of attacks were omitted from the tabulation. The results are shown in Tables 1 and 2.

TABLE 1. RECURRENCE OF ATTACKS IN MANIC-DEPRESSIVE MALE PATIENTS ADMITTED TO THE NEW YORK CIVIL STATE HOSPITALS, 1910 TO 1920

		NUMBER Number of attacks reported at last admission									
Type	Total	1	2	3	4	5	6	7	8	9	10 or more
Manic	1,762	967	456	159	81	39	21	14	8	4	13
Depressive ..	1,077	618	264	100	52	27	2	7	3	1	3
Mixed	280	156	73	24	16	5	1	..	2	1	2
Circular	128	73	30	12	6	3	1	1	..	2	..
Total	3,247	1,814	823	295	155	74	25	22	13	8	18
				PER CENT							
Manic	100.0	54.9	25.9	9.0	4.6	2.2	1.2	0.8	0.5	0.2	0.7
Depressive ..	100.0	57.4	24.5	9.3	4.8	2.5	0.2	0.6	0.3	0.1	0.3
Mixed	100.0	55.7	26.1	8.6	5.7	1.8	0.4	..	0.7	0.4	0.7
Circular	100.0	57.0	23.4	9.4	4.7	2.3	0.8	0.8	..	1.6	..
Total	100.0	55.9	25.3	9.1	4.8	2.3	0.8	0.7	0.4	0.2	0.6

TABLE 2. RECURRENCE OF ATTACKS IN MANIC-DEPRESSIVE FEMALE PATIENTS ADMITTED TO THE NEW YORK CIVIL STATE HOSPITALS, 1910 TO 1920

Type	Total	NUMBER Number of attacks reported at last admission 1	2	3	4	5	6	7	8	9	10 or more
Manic	2,548	1,420	617	260	124	56	28	16	5	5	17
Depressive ..	1,622	974	374	152	55	34	13	5	4	3	8
Mixed	845	506	205	76	34	12	4	2	2	1	3
Circular	176	102	41	14	7	5	3	3	..	..	1
Total	5,191	3,002	1,237	502	220	107	48	26	11	9	29
				PER CENT							
Manic	100.0	55.7	24.2	10.2	4.9	2.2	1.1	0.6	0.2	0.2	0.7
Depressive ..	100.0	60.0	23.1	9.4	3.4	2.1	0.8	0.3	0.2	0.2	0.5
Mixed	100.0	59.9	24.3	9.0	4.0	1.4	0.5	0.2	0.2	0.1	0.4
Circular	100.0	58.0	23.3	8.0	4.0	2.8	1.7	1.7	..	..	0.6
Total	100.0	57.8	23.8	9.7	4.2	2.1	0.9	0.5	0.2	0.2	0.6

Of the 3,247 males patients tabulated, 1,814, or 55.9 per cent, were reported as having had but one attack; 823, or 25.3 per cent, as having had but two attacks; 295, or 9.1 per cent, as having had but three attacks; 155, or 4.8 per cent, as having had but four attacks; 74, or 2.3 per cent, as having had but five attacks; and 86, or 2.7 per cent, as having had more than five attacks. The female cases that were ascertained with reference to type and number of attacks totaled 5,191. The percentage distribution by attacks were: Only one attack 57.8; only two attacks 23.8; only three attacks 9.7; only four attacks 4.2; only five attacks 2.1; more than five attacks 2.4. It will be noted that the relative frequency of attacks among females differs but little from that among males.

As the record of attacks tabulated covers only a part of the life history of the patients, the total attacks would be somewhat larger than the number indicated by these figures. The percentage of cases reported by Moore as having had but one attack was 27, and as having but two attacks 28. Macdonald found that 34.6 per cent of his cases had only one attack, and 65.4 per cent more than one.

In order to approach the matter from a different angle we tabulated the attacks and ages of the patients of the group studied that died in the hospital. The results are shown in Table 3.

TABLE 3. PER CENT DISTRIBUTION, BY AGE, OF ATTACKS OF THE MANIC-DEPRESSIVE PATIENTS STUDIED WHO DIED IN HOSPITAL

Age at death	Number of cases	Per cent distribution of attacks			
		1	2	3	More than 3
Under 20 years	53	81.2	16.7	2.1	...
20-24 years	141	81.3	15.7	2.2	0.7
25-29 years	136	76.7	18.6	4.7	...
30-34 years	150	73.1	17.7	7.0	2.1
35-39 years	141	68.2	20.9	6.2	4.7
40-44 years	135	58.7	31.7	5.6	4.0
45-49 years	158	53.3	30.0	12.7	4.0
50-54 years	137	49.6	32.0	11.2	7.2
55-59 years	109	40.0	32.4	13.3	14.3
60-64 years	91	35.4	36.6	15.9	12.2
65-69 years	68	26.2	45.9	14.8	13.1
70 years and over	77	21.1	25.4	23.9	29.6
Total	1,396*	58.1	26.1	9.3	6.5

*The distribution of attacks of 95 cases was unascertained.

Of the 1,301 deceased patients the number of whose attacks was ascertained, 736, or 58.1 per cent, died during the first attack; 340, or 26.1 per cent, during the second attack; 121, or 9.3 per cent, during the third attack; and 84, or 6.5 per cent, during subsequent attacks. The percentage of deaths of female patients occurring in the first attack was 60.8, and of the males 53.7.

Question 2.—*To what extent does the recurrence of attacks differ in the various types of manic-depressive psychoses?*

Of the 3,247 male cases tabulated, 1,762 were classified as of manic type; 1,077, as of depressive type; 280, as of mixed type; and 128, as of circular type. The number and percentage distribution of male cases by number of attacks for each type is shown in Table 1. The percentages of those having only one, only two, and only three attacks differ but little in the several types. The depressive type has the highest percentage of cases (57.4) having only one attack, and the manic type the lowest (54.9). The manic type has the largest percentage of cases having over five attacks.

Similar data for female cases are shown in Table 2. Of the 5,191 female cases tabulated, 2,548 were diagnosed as manic type; 1,622, as depressive type; 854, as mixed type; and 176, as circular type. Among females as among males, the manic type has the smallest percentage of cases having but one attack; the depressive type, on the other hand, has among both sexes the largest percentage of cases with only one attack. The differences in the per cent distribution of the cases of the various types classified by number of attacks are very small and indicate that type of reaction is not of great significance in relation to recurrence of attacks.

Question 3.—*How does the recurrence of attacks differ in the various age groups of first admissions?*

To answer this question we tabulated by age on admission and number of attacks reported at last admission, 1,703 cases comprising the first admissions of the fiscal years 1910, 1911 and 1912. The results are set forth in Table 4.

TABLE 4. PER CENT DISTRIBUTION OF ATTACKS OF 1,703 MANIC-DEPRESSIVE ADMISSIONS* TO THE NEW YORK CIVIL STATE HOSPITALS, CLASSIFIED BY AGE AT FIRST ADMISSION

Age at first admission	Total cases	Per cent distribution of attacks			
		1	2	3	More than 3
Under 20 years	209	52.2	25.8	11.0	11.0
20-24 years	307	67.1	19.0	8.8	5.2
25-29 years	235	62.6	18.3	11.1	8.1
30-34 years	213	59.1	20.2	11.7	8.9
35-39 years	190	58.9	19.5	8.9	12.6
40-44 years	158	47.5	28.5	12.7	11.4
45-49 years	134	43.3	23.9	11.2	21.6
50-54 years	100	47.0	28.0	13.0	12.0
55 years and over	157	52.9	22.3	14.6	10.2
Total	1,703	56.5	22.0	11.1	10.3

*First admissions of 1910, 1911 and 1912.

Of the group as a whole 56.5 per cent were reported as having had but one attack. The age groups from 20 to 40 years have higher percentages than the average of cases with one attack only. The other age groups have percentages lower than the average. In other words the patients between 20 and 40 years of age at time of first admission have fewer recurrences of attack than cases younger or older. Patients between 45 and 50 years of age at time of first admission have more attacks than those of other age groups.

Question 4.—*What is the average duration of attacks in manic-depressive psychoses?*

To answer this question we tabulated by age on discharge the 878 manic-depressive cases discharged as recovered in 1920. The results are shown in Table 5.

TABLE 5. AVERAGE DURATION, BY AGE, OF ATTACKS OF MANIC-DEPRESSIVE PATIENTS DISCHARGED AS RECOVERED FROM NEW YORK CIVIL STATE HOSPITALS, 1920

Age on discharge	Number of patients	Average duration of attacks in years					
		All attacks	First attack	Second attack	Third attack	Fourth attack	Fifth attack
Under 20 years	68	0.6	0.6	0.6	0.3	0.3	0.1
20-24 years	124	0.9	0.9	0.6	0.5	0.8	1.8
25-29 years	114	0.7	0.7	0.8	0.6	0.3	0.7
30-34 years	108	1.0	0.9	0.8	1.4	1.6	0.7
35-39 years	122	1.1	1.3	0.7	1.0	1.0	0.8
40-44 years	88	1.1	1.5	0.8	0.9	0.8	1.1
45-49 years	74	1.2	1.5	0.7	0.7	0.2	0.9
50-54 years	70	1.7	1.8	1.8	0.5	0.4	2.3
55-59 years	52	1.3	2.0	1.9	0.7	1.5	0.9
60-64 years	32	1.6	0.3	1.7	1.0	2.4	1.7
65-69 years	20	1.7	3.9	0.4	0.9	1.1	2.2
70 years and over	6	1.1	3.0	0.8	...	...	0.8
Total	878	1.1	1.1	1.0	0.9	0.9	1.2

The average duration of attacks among males was found to be 1.0 year and among females, 1.1 years. The average duration of first attacks among the former was 0.9 of a year and among the latter 1.3 years. Only slight variations from these periods are found for the other attacks.

With respect to age of patient it is noted that the duration of attack increases irregularly with advancing age.

It is, of course, realized that the average duration of attacks of recovered cases is shorter than that of all cases, but as many of the unrecovered cases are discharged as improved, it is almost impossible to ascertain the duration of their attacks.

Conclusions

1. Although manic-depressive psychoses are usually spoken of as recurrent forms of mental disease, it appears from these data that in more than half of the cases there is no recurrence of attack of sufficient severity to cause readmission to a hospital for mental disease.

2. The frequency of recurrence of attacks is nearly the same in the two sexes.

3. The frequency of recurrence of attacks differs but little in the various types of these psychoses.

4. Patients who are between 20 and 40 years of age at time of first admission have fewer recurrences of attacks than patients younger or older.

5. The average duration of attacks of recovered cases is a little more than one year. The average duration of successive attacks varies but little.

6. The average duration of attacks increases irregularly with advancing age.

CHAPTER VIII

Hereditary and Environmental Factors in the Causation of Manic-Depressive Psychoses and Dementia Præcox*

In 1928 the Laura Spelman Rockefeller Memorial made a grant to the State Charities Aid Association for a series of investigations into mental disease in New York State. The New York State Department of Mental Hygiene collaborated with the association in the investigations made. One line of research dealt with the prehospital histories of patients with mental disease. It was felt that such a study might clarify certain problems connected with the causation of mental disease. Social workers were therefore assigned to the Utica State Hospital and during the three years from 1928 to 1930 they conducted thorough investigations into the histories of two groups of patients admitted to that hospital. One group consisted of 155 first admissions with manic-depressive psychoses, of whom 60 were males and 95 females. The other consisted of 175 first admissions with dementia præcox, of whom 92 were males and 83 females. The patients were chosen for investigation in a random manner, there being no selective factor other than the existence of a well-defined psychosis. The Utica State Hospital was the locus of the investigation because its admission district includes a population easily accessible to investigation.

Information was obtained with respect to the mental and physical health of parents, grandparents, uncles, aunts and siblings of patients, special attention being directed to the occurrence of mental and nervous diseases, mental defect, alcoholism and criminality in the family stock. The information was gathered, whenever possible, through the direct testimony of the patient, close relatives and intimate associates. Interviews were held by the social workers at the hospital and in the field. All statements concerning the patient and his family were verified, whenever possible, through the direct testimony of first-hand sources; mere hearsay was avoided. Data were also gathered with respect to the developmental histories of the patients prior to the onset of the mental

*Read at the ninety-fifth annual meeting of The American Psychiatric Association, Chicago, Illinois, May 8-12, 1939.

For a fuller discussion of the subject, see the book entitled, "Hereditary and Environmental Factors in the Causation of Manic-Depressive Psychoses and Dementia Præcox," by Horatio M. Pollock, Benjamin Malzberg and Raymond G. Fuller, State Hospitals Press, Utica, N. Y., 1939.

disorder. These also related to the health of the patient at stated periods in his life. There was a description of the home life and of the relations between the patient and members of the household and of the character of the community in which he lived. The histories also included the school record, the occupational record, sex and marital experiences, etc.

In analyzing this mass of data, we began with the thesis that there is no known organic basis for either a manic-depressive psychosis or dementia præcox. Innumerable conditions have at one time or another been declared to be causative factors in these diseases, but laboratory investigations have always failed to confirm the claims. Our investigations were therefore directed to the study of two sets of factors. One is found in the familial histories of the patients; the other deals with the effects of certain biopsychological experiences upon the individual.

We start first with the family background. The analysis of such data has proceeded along two lines. According to one method, we assume the fact of inheritance and we attempt to fit the observations to a specified law of heredity. Agreement of the two is considered proof of inheritance. According to the second method we assume no law of heredity, but we search for differences in the incidence of tainting factors among the families of the mentally diseased and among a corresponding healthy population. If significant differences are found, it is assumed, that, other things being equal, they are due to the force of heredity.

The first method has proceeded along the lines of Mendelian analysis. Assuming, for example, that mental disease is a recessive character, the absence of mental disease being considered dominant, the parental generations are classified according to the presence or absence of mental disease. Now, on the assumption of Mendelian inheritance none of the parents of our patients should be classified as DD, for from the union of DD with DR or RR no diseased offspring should result. Parents who are outwardly normal must therefore be assumed to be of type DR. Mentally diseased parents must be considered of type RR. We must therefore consider the offspring resulting from the mating of DR with DR, of DR with RR, and of RR with RR. The first type should result in 25 per cent of the offspring being mentally diseased. From the second type of mating there should arise 50 per cent of diseased children. Progeny resulting from the third type of mating should all be mentally diseased.

TABLE 1. OFFSPRING OF PARENTS OF ASSUMED TYPE DR × DR, CLASSIFIED BY AGE AT DEATH OR AGE AT TIME OF ADMISSION OF THE PROBAND TO THE UTICA STATE HOSPITAL—MANIC-DEPRESSIVE STUDY

Age (years)	Deceased siblings*		Living siblings*	
	Number of cases	Number with mental disorder	Number of cases	Number with mental disorder
Under 10	57		1	
10-14	7		6	
15-19	4		11	
20-24	8		26	
25-29	3	1 general paresis	31	1 manic-depressive psychosis 1 dementia præcox
30-34	2		36	1 manic-depressive psychosis 1 unknown psychosis 1 psychopath
35-39	7	1 suicide	40	
40-44	5		38	1 nervous
45-49	4	1 general paresis	28	3 nervous 1 alcoholic
50-54	4	1 manic-depressive psychosis	37	1 feebleminded 1 nervous
55-59	2		22	2 nervous
60-64	..		13	
65-69	1		14	
70-74	..		5	
75-79	2		2	1 manic-depressive psychosis
Total	106	4	310	15

*Exclusive of proband.

Table 1 is based upon the histories of 82 patients with manic-depressive psychoses, and describes the siblings in those cases in which the parents were classified as DR × DR. In these families there should be mentally diseased offspring in the ratio of 1 diseased to 3 normal. There were 416 children, exclusive of the probands. On Mendelian theory there should therefore have been

104±6.0 diseased children. By defining mental disease as widely as possible, and by including such conditions as suicide, nervousness, depression, etc., as indications of a neuropathic taint, we obtain a total of 19 cases of mental disease. This is only 22 per cent of the minimum required on the hypothesis that mental disease is a recessive unit character. As age is an important complicating factor, several corrections were made, but in no case was it possible to obtain agreement with the requirements of Mendelian theory.

The hypothesis of DR × RR was tested in connection with 48 families. There were 230 siblings, exclusive of the probands. Half, or 115, should have been mentally diseased. Actually there were only 31 such cases, including 1 case of general paresis, 6 of manic-depressive psychoses, 1 of involution melancholia, 4 of dementia præcox, 2 unknown psychoses, 1 case of epilepsy, 7 cases of nervousness, 2 suicides, and 7 cases of alcoholism. Corrections for age did not bring about any significant changes in the results.

Finally, we may consider 8 families in which the matings were of the variety RR × RR. In 3 of these, the matings may be considered strictly of this type, since both parents were either feebleminded or mentally diseased. In the remaining 5 families, the matings represented unions of 2 nervous individuals, of a nervous individual with an alcoholic, and of an alcoholic with an alcoholic. On the assumption that these are of the same value from the Mendelian point of view, all the offspring should have been mentally diseased. There were 35 siblings, exclusive of the probands. Of these, only 9 were affected, of whom 8 were feebleminded, and 1 was a case of manic-depressive psychosis. The total is too small for significant comparison, but it is noteworthy, nevertheless, that once again fact and theory were not in agreement.

We turn next to dementia præcox. Table 2 considers 101 families in which both parents were described as normal and who must therefore be classified as latent dominants. In these families there were 458 siblings, exclusive of the 101 probands. There were 26 affected siblings, including 6 with psychoses, 4 alcoholics, 7 nervous, 2 suicides, 2 neurotic, 4 feebleminded and 1 epileptic. There should have been 114.5±6.3 cases of affected siblings. The actual total was thus far less than the minimum expected on the basis of random sampling.

TABLE 2. OFFSPRING OF PARENTS OF ASSUMED TYPE DR × DR, CLASSIFIED BY AGE AT DEATH OR AGE AT TIME OF ADMISSION OF THE PROBAND TO THE UTICA STATE HOSPITAL—DEMENTIA PRÆCOX STUDY

Age (years)	Deceased siblings*		Living siblings*	
	Number of cases	Number with mental disorder	Number of cases	Number with mental disorder
Under 10	50		9	
10-14	5		19	1 feebleminded
15-19	2		31	1 nervous
20-24	11		31	
25-29	8	1 alcoholic	44	
30-34	6	1 nervous	41	1 neurotic 1 nervous
35-39	2	1 suicide	56	1 alcoholic 3 feebleminded 1 nervous 1 unknown psychosis
40-44	3		42	2 nervous 2 alcoholic 1 epileptic
45-49	1		35	4 unknown psychoses
50-54	3	1 neurotic	24	
55-59	2	1 suicide	10	
60-64	2		5	
65-69	..		6	1 nervous 1 dementia præcox
70-74	..		2	
75-79	1		2	
Unknown	5†		..	
Total	101	5	357	21

*Exclusive of proband.

†All under 50 years of age.

In 47 families the matings were considered of the type DR × RR. The offspring totaled 165, exclusive of the probands. Of the siblings, 16 were classified as mentally tainted. On a Mendelian basis there should have been 82.5±4.3 such cases. Clearly, there is no agreement between fact and theory.

Finally, there was a series of 14 families in which both parents were tainted. In these families there were 66 children, exclusive of the probands. Among them were 5 cases of feeblemindednss, 1 of dementia præcox, and 1 of nervousness, a total of 7. According to the theory, all 66 should have been mentally diseased.

We conclude therefore that neither dementia præcox nor manic-depressive psychoses appears in frequencies that are in accord with the requirements of simple Mendelian inheritance. It has been suggested by several investigators that the hypothesis of dihybridism would give an adequate explanation of the frequency of certain types of mental diseases. But if we complicate hypotheses, it may always be possible to obtain concordance between fact and theory. However, such agreement cannot be the only criterion. One must seek underlying reasons justifying the application of a particular formula.

Search for such justification, however, only increases the distrust in the possibility of applying Mendelian laws to the inheritance of mental disease. In the first place, there should be clear-cut clinical entities with respect to the several types of mental disorders. We should, for example, study the offspring of parents who were dominant or recessive with respect to manic-depressive psychoses or dementia præcox. Among the offspring, there should be found individuals affected with such psychoses in ratios required by Mendelian theory. We have already shown that this requirement could not be met in our family data. In the second place, the development of the mental disorders should be independent of external circumstances. If this is not the case, we cannot hope to obtain the correct total of recessives, for it is conceivable that under a favorable environment no one might develop a mental disease. How different is the case with such characters as eye color, for example, where the trait appears in a constant proportion among the offspring, independently of environmental changes other than those of a pathological order, that may affect the entire organism. In the third place, there should be no differential mortality between the several genotypes. If those with the diathesis for a manic-depressive psychosis, for example, have higher rates of infant and child mortality than the normal children, then the frequency of appearance of the disease would be less than the minimum requirements of Mendelian theory. Finally, are we justified in assuming that a mental disease may be treated as a unit, the transmission of which through inheritance is independent of the transmission of other characters? Is it not at least conceivable that there is correlation instead of independence of mental traits, and that the frequency of a mental disorder is therefore in part a function of the nature of the organism as a whole?

Thus far we have failed to establish the existence of a particular form of inheritance, but this does not necessitate the inference that heredity is not a factor in the origin and transmission of mental disorders. We must observe the frequencies of mental disease in the families of the patients, and compare them with frequencies in other populations. The first investigations of this type were reported by Koller and Diem. Both found higher percentages of individuals with so-called tainting factors in the families of patients with mental disease than among the families of healthy individuals, though the differences were smaller than had been anticipated. In recent years Rüdin and his associates in Munich have attempted to arrive at samples of the normal population through a consideration of the spouses of patients with general paresis or with cerebral arteriosclerosis. The selection of the spouses was made on the assumption that, since these disorders are presumably on a nonhereditary basis, the presence of the disease in husband or wife will not have been of genetic, significance in the inheritance of the marital partner. However, it is unlikely that a satisfactory sample of a normal population (adequate in size and randomness of choice) can be secured for the purpose of comparison with the families of mental patients. The selective factors operating to vitiate the random choice of samples of a general population are extremely subtle, and one can hardly ever be certain that such factors have not entered into the choice of a numerically limited sample.

We may, however, proceed in the following manner. By means of our family histories we are able to count the total number of relatives of specified degree, and the corresponding numbers of affected individuals. The proportion of affected individuals may then be compared with the corresponding proportion for the general population. If each class formed only a random sample of the general population, the proportions of affected individuals should not differ sensibly from that of the general population.

In such an analysis it is necessary to know the expectation of mental disease. Under given conditions of mortality it is required to know how many in a given generation will develop mental disease in the course of a life time. This expectation has been determined for New York State, where it was found that, in 1920, males had a chance of 4.7 in 100 of developing a mental disorder, females 4.4 in 100. On the theory of random sampling, approximately 4.7 per cent of male populations and 4.4 per cent of female populations should therefore develop mental disease. These may be called "crude" expectations for the families of the patients, however, since the assumptions underlying the expectations for 1920 cannot be applied directly to those of the older generations. The expectations for 1920 are the result of rates of mental disease and rates of mortality in that year. Both sets of rates have been subject to a secular trend. The rate of mental disease has been increasing from decade to decade and general mortality rates have been decreasing. Twenty and 40 years ago admission rates were decidedly lower than they are today, whereas death rates were materially higher. Consequently, the expectation of mental disease in the several older generations must have been less than 4.7 per cent and 4.4 per cent, for males and females, respectively. The grandparental generation included the period from 1820 to 1900; the parental generation and the collaterals included a period from approximately 1850 to 1930. The siblings embrace the period beginning at about 1890. Considering the changes in death rates and rates of mental disease it appears conservative to estimate, in comparison with the expectations of 1920, an average expectation of 4.0 for males and 3.5 for females throughout the earlier periods. Applications of such corrected expectations to the families of the patients will give figures legitimately comparable with the recorded findings.

The principal data are shown in Tables 3 and 4 for the families of the patients with manic-depressive psychoses. It will be noted that there were 2,572 relatives in the histories. No details were recorded in 195 cases, leaving a total of 2,377 with recorded histories. Among the latter there were 58 with mental diseases.

The total of recorded psychoses is undoubtedly too low. This is due in part to the fact that in each degree of relationship there are individuals still exposed to the chance of developing a mental disorder. We may compensate for this by applying the appropriate expectations of mental disease. We cannot compensate, however, for the incomplete histories of many of the patients. Not all were native-born with families easily accessible to investigation by the

TABLE 3. FREQUENCY OF MENTAL DISORDERS AMONG THE RELATIVES OF 155 PATIENTS WITH MANIC-DEPRESSIVE PSYCHOSES

Relationship	Total number of relatives	No details recorded	Number of histories recorded	Total without mental disease or other specified defect	Totals: Number with psychoses	Totals: Number with other defects	Totals: Total defects or diseases recorded*	Psychoses: Senile psychosis	Psychoses: With cerebral arteriosclerosis	Psychoses: General paresis	Psychoses: Alcoholic psychoses	Psychoses: Manic-depressive	Psychoses: Involution melancholia	Psychoses: Dementia præcox	Psychoses: Epileptic psychoses	Psychoses: Psychoneuroses	Psychoses: Undiagnosed psychoses	Other defects: Neurotic traits	Other defects: Mental deficiency	Other defects: Epilepsy	Other defects: Alcoholism	Other defects: Drug addiction	Other defects: Suicide
Father	155	1	154	115	3	36	41	..	..	..	..	3	..	..	..	..	..	13	1	1	19	..	4
Mother	155	1	154	122	6	26	36	..	1	..	..	1	..	2	..	..	2	25	2	..	2	1	..
Paternal grandfather	155	34	121	115	3	3	9	..	..	..	..	1	..	..	..	..	2	..	..	..	5	..	1
Paternal grandmother	155	37	118	115	1	2	3	..	..	..	..	..	..	..	..	..	1	2	..	..	..	..	..
Maternal grandfather	155	29	126	123	1	2	3	..	..	..	..	..	..	..	..	..	1	..	..	..	..	..	2
Maternal grandmother	155	26	129	125	1	3	4	..	..	..	..	..	..	..	..	..	1	3	..	..	..	..	..
Paternal uncles	229	17	212	201	5	6	11	1	..	..	1	..	..	..	..	..	3	..	..	1	5	..	..
Paternal aunts	187	12	175	171	2	2	4	..	..	..	..	..	..	..	..	..	2	1	..	1	..	..	..
Maternal uncles	228	10	218	210	2	6	9	..	..	..	..	1	..	1	..	..	..	..	..	..	6	..	1
Maternal aunts	231	6	225	217	5	3	8	..	..	..	..	1	..	..	..	..	4	2	..	1	..	..	..
Brothers	380	11	369	333	15	21	36	..	..	3	1	3	..	5	1	..	2	7	5	..	7	..	2
Sisters	387	11	376	346	14	16	32	..	..	1	..	7	1	2	..	1	2	11	3	1	..	..	3
Total	2,572	195	2,377	2,193	58	126	196	1	1	4	2	17	1	10	1	1	20	64	11	5	44	1	13

*An individual may have more than one defect.

TABLE 4. COMPARISON OF EXPECTED WITH CORRECTED TOTAL OF ACTUAL CASES OF MENTAL DISEASE IN THE FAMILIES OF 155 PATIENTS WITH MANIC-DEPRESSIVE PSYCHOSES

Relationship	Number with known histories	Expected cases of mental disease	Actual cases of mental disease	Anticipated cases
Father	154	6.2	3	1.6
Mother	154	5.4	6	1.8
Paternal grandfather	121	4.9	3	...
Paternal grandmother	118	4.1	1	0.2
Maternal grandfather	126	5.1	1	...
Maternal grandmother	129	4.6	1	0.2
Paternal uncles	212	8.5	5	2.1
Paternal aunts	175	6.1	2	2.1
Maternal uncles	218	8.7	2	3.0
Maternal aunts	225	7.9	5	2.7
Brothers	369	14.8	15	11.0
Sisters	376	13.2	14	11.2
Total	2,377	89.5	58	35.9

field workers. Many histories were therefore based on incomplete evidence, and it is not beyond the bounds of reasonable probability that they include individuals who should be added to the total cases of mental disease. These errors will be apparent with respect to the ancestral generations, where it is shown in the accompanying table that the expected cases of mental disease are in excess of the actual plus anticipated cases, except for the mothers. Among the siblings, however, for whom the information is much more reliable, we find a total of 369 brothers and 376 sisters with known histories. Among the former there were 15 cases of mental disease, and a further anticipation of 11 cases, a total of 26, compared with an expectation of only 14.8. Among the sisters there were 14 known cases of mental diseases, and an anticipation of 11.2 cases, making a total of 25.2, compared with a complete expectation of only 13.2 cases. Clearly, among the siblings, for whom the data are most adequate, there is an excess of mental disorders over the total expected in a random sample.

There were 39 families in which a father had a mental disease or some defect usually considered a tainting factor. In these 39 families there were, exclusive of the probands, 112 brothers and 85 sisters with adequate histories. The brothers included 4 known cases of mental disease, and an anticipation of 2.7 cases, a total of 6.7, compared with a complete expectation of 4.5 cases. The sisters included 4 known cases of mental disease, with an anticipation of 2.0 additional cases, a total of 6.0, compared with a complete expectation of 3.0.

Thirty-two mothers were described as tainted. In these families there were 80 brothers and 65 sisters with adequate histories. Among the brothers there were 6 known cases of mental disease, with an anticipation of 2.2 cases, a total of 8.2, compared with a complete expectation of 3.2. Among the sisters there were 5 known cases of mental disease, with an anticipation of 2.0 cases, a total of 7.0, compared with a complete expectation of only 2.3 cases.

There were 9 families in which both parents were tainted. In these families the siblings were too few in number, however, to give significant results. There were 24 brothers, among whom there was 1 case of mental disease, and an anticipation of 0.4, a total of 1.4, compared with an expectation of 1.0. There were 19 sisters who included 1 case of mental disease and an anticipation of 0.4, a total of 1.4, compared with an expectation of 0.7 cases.

Finally, we may consider the frequency of manic-depressive psychoses among the siblings of patients with manic-depressive psychoses. The latter had 369 brothers and 376 sisters. Among the former there were 3 cases of manic-depressive psychoses, and an anticipation of 1.0 case, a total of 4.0, compared with a complete expectation of 1.8 cases. Among the sisters there were 7 cases of manic-depressive psychoses, and an anticipation of 2.9 cases, a total of 9.9, compared with an expectation of only 3.4 cases.

We shall next consider the incidence of mental disease among the families of the patients with dementia præcox. The necessary data are included in Tables 5 and 6.

The family histories included 2,753 relatives, exclusive of the probands. The details were insufficient in 238 cases, leaving a total of 2,515 individuals with adequately recorded histories. Among the latter were 74 psychotic individuals. With proper consideration of the age factor, we should add 47.5 cases, making a total of 121.5, compared with a complete expectation of only 94.6. Because of their accessibility to investigation, the results for the siblings were more reliable. Among the brothers there were 11 with known

TABLE 5. FREQUENCY OF MENTAL DISORDERS AMONG THE RELATIVES OF 175 PATIENTS WITH DEMENTIA PRÆCOX

Relationship	Total number of relatives	No details recorded	Number of histories recorded	Total without mental disease or other specified defect	Totals: Number of psychoses	Totals: Number with other defects	Totals: Total defects or diseases recorded*	Psychoses: Senile psychoses	Psychoses: With cerebral arteriosclerosis	Psychoses: General paresis	Psychoses: Alcoholic psychosis	Psychoses: With other somatic diseases	Psychoses: Manic-depressive	Psychoses: Involution melancholia	Psychoses: Dementia præcox	Psychoses: Paranoia or paranoic conditions	Psychoses: Epileptic psychoses	Psychoses: Psychoneuroses and neuroses	Psychoses: With psychopathic personality	Psychoses: With mental deficiency	Psychoses: Undiagnosed psychoses	Other defects: Neurotic traits	Other defects: Mental deficiency	Other defects: Epilepsy	Other defects: Alcoholism	Other defects: Suicide
Father	175	1	174	133	4	37	47	..	..	..	..	..	2	..	2	..	..	..	..	..	..	11	1	..	30	1
Mother	175	1	174	128	13	33	46	1	..	..	..	1	3	..	4	..	..	..	..	..	4	32	1	..	..	..
Paternal grandfather ..	175	40	135	123	2	10	14	..	..	..	..	..	1	..	..	1	..	..	..	..	..	3	..	..	8	1
Paternal grandmother .	175	40	135	127	5	3	8	1	..	..	..	..	1	..	..	..	..	..	..	..	3	3	..	..	..	..
Maternal grandfather ..	175	41	134	122	5	7	13	1	..	1	..	..	1	..	..	..	..	..	..	..	2	1	..	..	6	1
Maternal grandmother .	175	38	137	136	1	..	1	..	..	..	..	..	..	1	..	..	..	..	..	..	..	..	..	..	..	..
Paternal uncles.	259	22	237	215	6	16	26	..	1	..	1	1	..	..	2	..	..	..	..	..	1	2	..	..	16	2
Paternal aunts..	211	11	200	189	4	7	11	..	..	..	..	..	1	..	2	..	..	..	..	1	..	6	1	..	..	..
Maternal uncles.	254	12	242	223	7	12	22	..	..	..	..	..	4	..	..	..	1	..	1	..	1	1	3	..	9	2
Maternal aunts..	245	14	231	222	5	4	10	..	..	..	..	..	1	..	..	..	..	1	..	..	3	3	..	1	..	1
Brothers	381	7	374	346	11	17	28	1	1	..	..	..	..	..	4	..	..	..	..	1	4	4	5	..	6	2
Sisters	353	11	342	309	11	22	34	1	2	..	..	..	2	..	3	1	..	..	..	..	2	16	4	1	2	..
Total	2,753	238	2,515	2,273	74	168	260	5	4	1	1	2	16	1	17	2	1	1	1	2	20	82	15	2	77	10

*An individual may have more than one defect.

psychoses, and an anticipation of 12.7 additional cases, a total of 23.7, compared with an expectation of only 15.0 cases. Among the sisters there were 11 known cases of mental disease and an anticipation of 11.4 cases, a total of 22.4, compared with an expectation of only 12.0.

TABLE 6. COMPARISON OF EXPECTED WITH CORRECTED TOTAL OF ACTUAL CASES OF MENTAL DISEASE IN THE FAMILIES OF 175 PATIENTS WITH DEMENTIA PRÆCOX

Relationship	Number with known histories	Expected cases of mental disease	Actual known cases of mental disease	Anticipated cases
Father	174	7.0	4	2.4
Mother	174	6.1	13	2.8
Paternal grandfather	135	5.4	2	0.2
Paternal grandmother	135	4.7	5	0.4
Maternal grandfather	134	5.3	5	0.2
Maternal grandmother	137	4.8	1	0.7
Paternal uncles	237	9.5	6	4.5
Paternal aunts	200	7.0	4	3.5
Maternal uncles	242	9.7	7	4.5
Maternal aunts	231	8.1	5	4.2
Brothers	374	15.0	11	12.7
Sisters	342	12.0	11	11.4
Total	2,515	94.6	74	47.5

We may next consider the frequencies of mental disorders among the siblings under specified conditions of mental tainting among the parents.

In 27 families the father was tainted. In these families there were 114 siblings, exclusive of the 27 probands, consisting of 55 brothers and 59 sisters. Among the brothers there were 3 psychoses, and an anticipation of 2.0, a total of 5.0, whereas the expectation was only 2.2. Among the sisters there were 3 psychoses, and an anticipation of 1.8, giving a total of 4.8, compared with an expectation of 2.1.

In 32 families the mother was tainted. In these families there were 49 brothers and 44 sisters, exclusive of the probands. Among the brothers there were 2 psychoses, and an anticipation of 1.9 cases, a total of 3.9, compared with an expectation of 2.0. Among the sisters there were 4 psychoses, and an anticipation of 1.5, a total of 5.5, compared with an expectation of only 1.9.

There were 14 cases in which both parents were tainted. In these families there were 32 brothers and 34 sisters, exclusive of the probands. Because of the small totals the results cannot be considered significant. Among the brothers there was 1 psychosis, and an anticipation of 1.7, a total of 2.7, compared with an expectation of 1.3. Among the sisters there were no actual cases of psychoses. Those still exposed to a mental disease provided an anticipation of 1.2 cases, which is the same as the general expectation.

We shall consider, finally, the frequency of dementia præcox. Among the 374 brothers with known histories there were 4 cases of dementia præcox, with an anticipation of 4.2 cases, giving a total of 8.2, compared with an expectation of only 5.2. Among the 342 sisters there were 3 cases of dementia præcox, and an anticipation of 3.7, a total of 6.7, compared with an expectation of 4.2.

On the basis of family statistics of mental disease, we are now in a position to say that, though no specific law of inheritance of mental diseases has yet been proven, it does seem highly probable that there is a generalized familial basis for such disorders. The chance of developing a mental disorder is greater in such families than the corresponding chance for the general population.

Nevertheless, it would be a mistaken inference from the preceding data that a family predisposition, constitutional in nature, is an all-sufficient basis for the development of these mental disorders. The transmission of a mental disease from generation to generation is not a fatalistic process. The elements in the development of a mental disorder are not comparable to physical units which determine such characters as eye color or type of hair. The latter, so far as known, are the consequences of rigid and invariable laws, and appear at stated periods in the physiological development of the individual. Not so, however, are the facts with respect to mental disease. There is no evidence that mental disorders appear inevitably at certain life epochs with the regularity of physiological cycles. No one appears fated to develop dementia præcox because some ancestor had such a disease. It requires something in addition to a diathesis or predisposition. There must be not only a seed but a ground in which to plant the seed. Inferior human stock may still be enabled, through proper nurture, to achieve a life of a fair degree of usefulness. On the other hand, we know that even the soundest of stock may succumb to the repeated onslaught of an unfavorable environment.

We conclude, therefore, that we cannot speak of hereditary and environmental factors as antithetic causes of mental disease. Both combine, often in subtle ways, to create such disorders. Persons with a diathesis for mental disease will undoubtedly succumb readily to many environmental stresses, which others, more fortunate in their family endowment, may be able to resist and overcome. But certain stresses are of such intensity that if repeated at sufficient length they may overcome the resistance of even the soundest constitutions. It must, furthermore, be borne in mind that siblings are affected by like environmental influences during their formative years. If faulty family habits, attitudes or conditions are factors in causing the mental breakdown of the probands, is it not probable that they would also unfavorably affect some of the other siblings? In the single family circle there is a blending of hereditary and environmental factors that renders it difficult to evaluate their respective influences on the development and health of the children.

In addition to inheritance or family background we must therefore consider two other elements, namely, the personality and the environment. Personality, though sometimes the result of inherited traits, usually develops to a great extent apart from such influences. More significant appears to be the psychic environment into which one is born and in which one grows up. The environment acts directly upon the mind through various types of stimuli, and it arouses the imitative processes. Environment also acts indirectly by encouraging the selection of traits. Thus, directly and indirectly, the environment brings about the various combinations which form the human personality. Some of these traits are correlated with unhealthy mental trends, and may be recognized in what Dr. August Hoch called the "shut-in" personality. The chief characteristics of the latter are the possession of a seclusive disposition and the gradual withdrawal of such persons from social contacts. This, in extreme cases, gives rise to certain types of reaction, emphasized by Dr. Adolf Meyer, which, if maintained over long periods of time, may result in abnormal behavior. We thus have a fusion of psychological and biological elements into the formation of a diseased personality. The process is fairly clear among the patients with dementia præcox. A large percentage exhibited well-marked seclusive traits. These traits appeared to be encouraged as a result of extremely restricted social lives of the patients and their families. A high percentage of these families were described as having no social contacts with persons outside the restricted family limits. As they grew older, the patients demonstrated lack of a normal degree of aggressive and adventurous spirit by failure to strike out for themselves and to create new careers and new homes. A surprisingly high percentage failed to marry, and of those who did many failed to adjust and their marriages landed on rocky shores. In their economic activities many were failures in obtaining and in holding jobs. In a high percentage of the families there was a distinct lowering of economic status as the patients grew from childhood to manhood.

Among the manic-depressives we also found abnormal trends in personality, but in addition to seclusiveness, we found depressiveness, instability and overactivity. These mental characteristics were played upon by environmental forces until the breaking point was reached with respect to individual strength. Lowered physical resistance seems to play a significant part, whereby adverse circumstances which might otherwise be overcome cannot be borne. If we analyze those situations existing just prior to the mental breakdown, we find frequent references to financial difficulties, worry over death or sickness, and sex difficulties and disappointments. But merely because these precede the mental illness, it would be dangerous to infer that they are sufficient causes. Rather we seem justified in concluding that situations which may be of no significance to persons in otherwise sound health may prove decisive factors among those who are weakened by constitutional factors or physical disease.

If the immediate exciting factors in manic-depressive psychoses and dementia præcox are compared, it will be noted that there are no essential differences. The factors are not specific. Evidently, therefore, the type of mental disease depends primarily upon the nature of the organism upon which these external forces play. Persons who develop a manic-depressive psychosis must differ in essential traits from those who develop dementia præcox. What these differences arise from is still largely unknown. It is possible that light may be cast upon the psychological processes in these mental disorders through a fuller understanding of the newer results being obtained from the application of insulin therapy. Used originally in connection with dementia præcox, hypoglycemic shock has also been used upon manic-depressive patients, and some startling results in therapy have been observed in both groups. Psychiatrists are beginning to study the psychological changes that accompany the processes of recovery, and it is possible that by reversing the approach they may obtain a valuable insight into the formation of those psychological trends which originally brought about the diseased mental condition.

Mental disease is a tragedy to the individual and his family, and a burden to society. It is important, therefore, that encouragement be given to all forms of research which may ultimately throw light upon the nature of mental disorders. We need more, not less, investigation into brain anatomy and physiology. We need additional studies into the nature of hereditary influences. Studies into the relation of constitution to disease should be carried out in greater detail. But we also need a better understanding of how human beings are molded by their environments. From a synthesis of such fields of research there will some day come a more adequate conception of the causative factors in mental disease.

CHAPTER IX

Mental Disease in the United States in Relation to Environment, Sex and Age, 1922*

Through the courtesy of the director of the Federal Census Bureau, I am privileged to present important data compiled for the report of the census of hospitals for mental disease taken January 1, 1923. This census included the patients resident in hospitals on such date and the first admissions, readmissions, discharges and deaths for the year 1922. Altogether 526 institutions for mental disease were represented, of which 163 were state hospitals, 2 government hospitals, 148 other public hospitals, and 213 private institutions. The resident patients numbered 267,617 and those on parole or temporarily absent from the institutions, 22,839. The patients received by the institutions in 1922 included 73,063 first admissions, 16,392 readmissions, and 4,607 transfers. The departures from the institutions comprised 52,777 discharges, 4,731 transfers, and 25,556 deaths. Individual schedules for each of the movement groups were received from every state hospital, except that of Montana, and from nearly all of the private institutions.

This study is based on 63,624 first admissions whose environment, sex and age were reported on uniform schedules filled out by the employees of the hospitals engaged by the Federal Census Bureau for such purpose. Cases unascertained with respect to environment are not considered.

Thanks to the activities of the Committee on Statistics of this Association,* the schedules included a caption calling for the mental classification of each patient. The data tabulated as a result of the census therefore not only sets forth facts concerning the patients of these institutions as a single class, but also data relating to each of the 22 clinical groups of the association's classification. This greatly enhances the value of the census.

It may be an agreeable form of mental exercise to talk and compile figures about the insane as a homogenous class, but the value of such data is very limited. The patients of the several clinical groups have little in common except that they live in the same type

*Read at the eighty-first annual meeting of The American Psychiatric Association, Richmond, Va., May 12, 13, 14, 15, 1925.

of institution, and knowledge of the characteristics of the so-called insane as a single group throws little light on the characteristics of the patients of any one psychosis. The charts to which I shall shortly refer show clearly that each of the principal groups of psychoses has its characteristic age and sex curve and that these curves vary widely from one another. The several groups also vary widely with respect to symptoms, prognosis, expectation of life, and duration of hospital life. In other words they are, in the main, separate disease entities and should be treated as such, both medically and statistically.

It is of course recognized that strict lines of demarcation cannot be drawn between some of the functional groups, but it is believed that fairly satisfactory uniformity in classifying the several groups has been attained.

In this series of charts we are dealing with rates of first admissions to institutions for mental disease from urban and rural communities in the United States, the rates in each instance being based on the general population of the same environment, sex and age. Cities and villages having a population of 2,500 or over are considered as urban and all other places as rural. Each chart contains four curves which show relative rates for urban males, urban females, rural males and rural females, respectively.

Chart 1 includes the whole group of 63,624 cases and shows in condensed form rates for first admissions to institutions for mental disease in 1922.

It will be noted that the rate of first admissions under 15 years of age is very small for each group. As adult life is reached the rates rapidly increase; they also rapidly diverge. During the middle period of life the increase with advancing age becomes less marked, but in the years of old age is again accelerated. Comparing the curves for males and females of urban and rural environment we note that urban males have the highest rate of first admissions in each age group. Urban females have the next highest rate in each age period except that of 20 to 24 years. Rural males have higher rates than rural females in every period except that of 50 to 54 years. Rural females have the lowest rates of all. The general average rates for all ages combined in the several groups are as follows: Urban males, 89.6; urban females, 67.8; rural males, 46.4; rural females, 35.5. When we behold these curves we can but regret the many unearned tears we have shed for the "poor, lonesome, languishing, isolated, farmer's wife."

In the succeeding charts you will observe how widely the curves for the separate groups vary from the general curves shown in Chart 1.

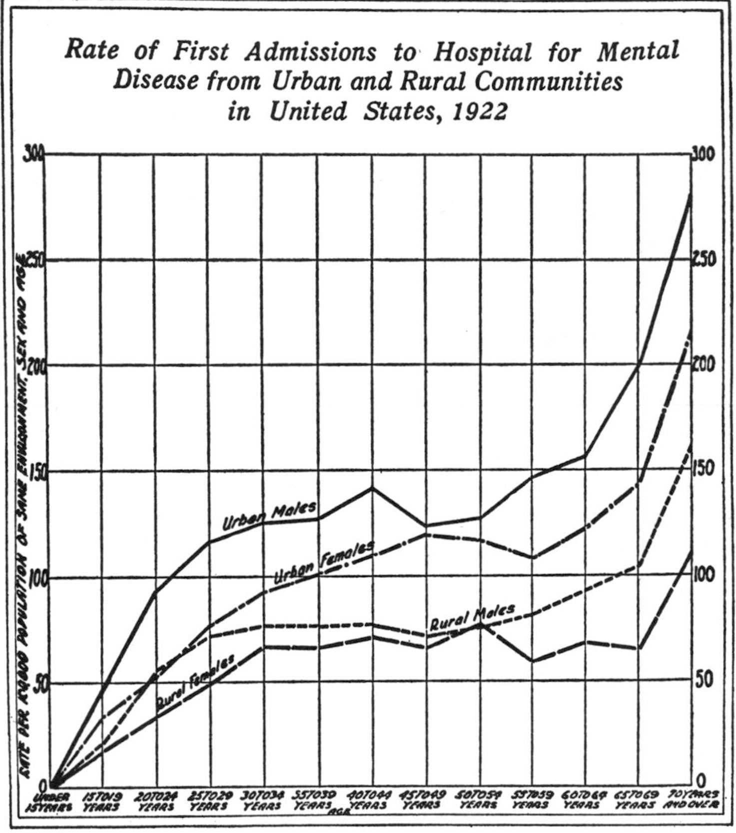

CHART I.

Chart 2 deals with 5,927 senile cases. Patients with senile psychoses, as the term implies, constitute an advanced age group, there being but few under 55 years of age. The rate of senile psychoses naturally increases rapidly from 60 years of age upward. The general average rate of senile psychoses in cities is higher among women than among men, the rates being 34.3 and 29.4, respectively. In the separate age groups the women have a higher rate in each group below 70 years. In rural districts the rate of senile psychoses is higher among men than among women, the general average rates being 23.1 and 20.3, respectively. In the age groups below 70 years, the rates in the two sexes vary but little, but in the group from 70 years and over the rate for men is 103.7 as compared to 80.3 for women.

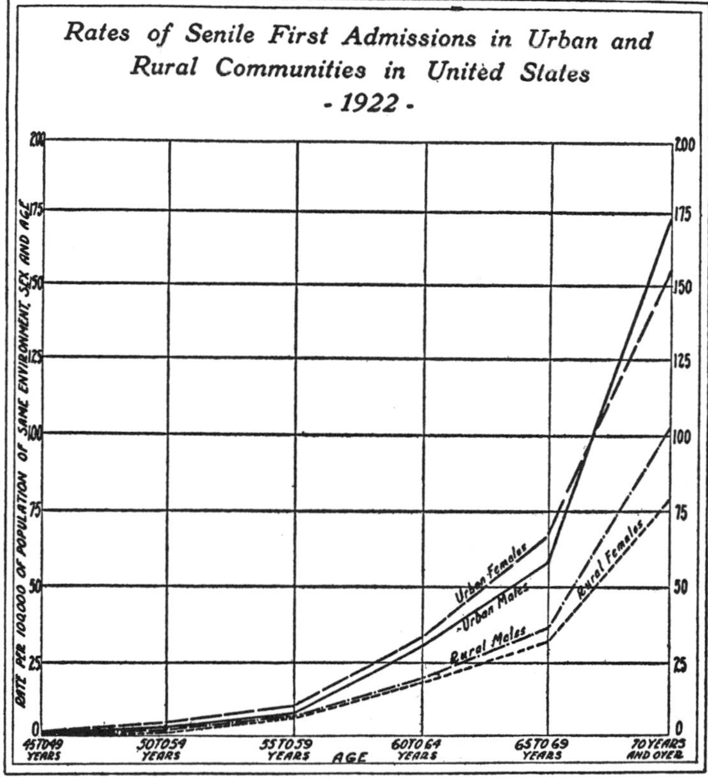

CHART 2.

Chart 3 comprises 3,006 cerebral arteriosclerotic cases. Psychoses with cerebral arteriosclerosis are also diseases of advanced life. In these psychoses the rates of first admissions are higher in cities than in rural districts and among males than among females. The rate for urban males is remarkably high compared with the rate for rural males. The rate for urban females in the earlier age groups is somewhat higher than that for rural males, but falls below the latter in the age group 65 to 69 years. The rates for rural females are the lowest in every life period. The general average rates in this psychosis are: Urban males, 21.1; urban females, 13.6; rural males, 12.4; rural females, 6.3.

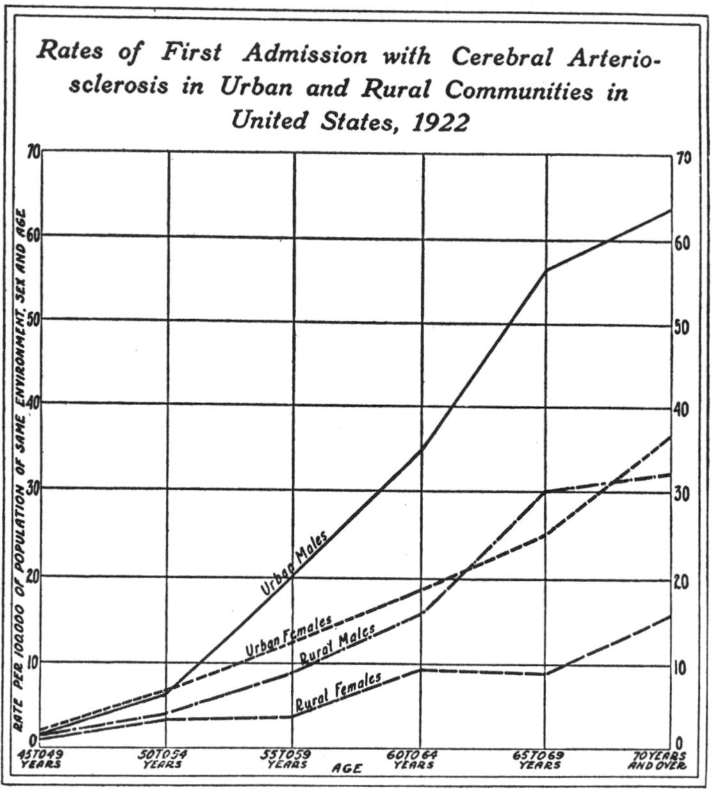

CHART 3.

Chart 4 deals with 5,515 cases of general paralysis. Here we are dealing with a disease that has its onset principally in middle life. As seen by this chart it is mainly a disorder affecting men in cities, the number of cases among urban men being nearly twice as great as the combined total of cases occurring among urban women and among rural men and women. The rate of first admissions among urban males is insignificant prior to age 25, but from that age upwards the rate increases with remarkable rapidity until the maximum is reached in the age period of 40 to 44 years. The rate remains at practically the same level until 50 years of age when it undergoes a rapid decline. The curve for rural males also reaches

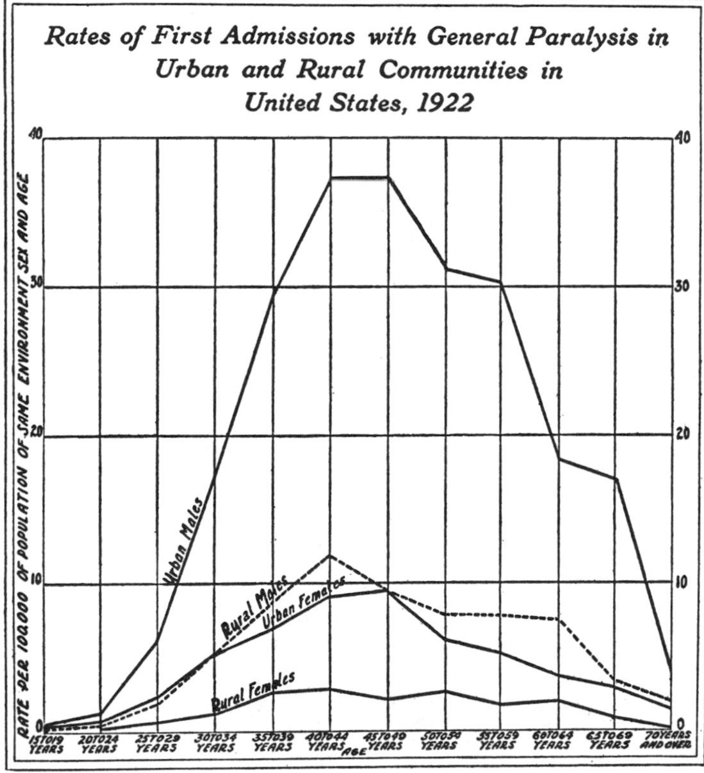

CHART 4.

its peak at the age of 40 to 44 years and then irregularly declines. The curve for urban females reaches its peak in age period 45 to 49 years. The curve for rural females is relatively insignificant. The general average rates in this psychosis are: Urban males, 18.3; urban females, 4.4; rural males, 5.1; rural females, 1.3. The special attention of health officers in cities is called to the results shown in this chart.

Chart 5 includes 2,337 first admissions with alcoholic psychoses. It indicates to a considerable degree the respect in which the Vol-

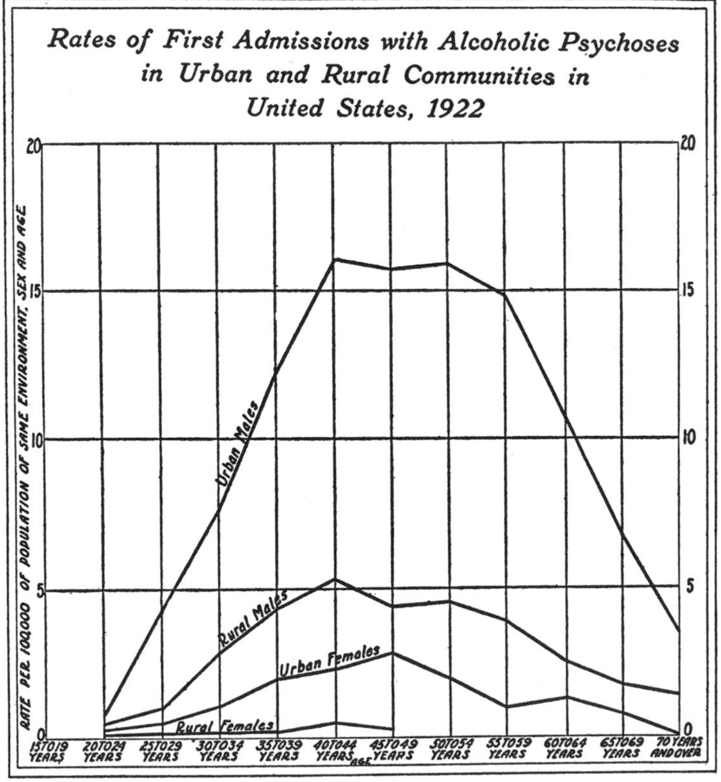

CHART 5.

stead Act was held by the groups represented by the curves. The predominance of alcoholism among males stands out prominently and it is probable that the higher rates in cities reflect the freer use of alcohol therein. There were only 20 alcoholic women admitted to hospitals for mental disease from rural districts in 1922. These were probably suburbanites. The curve for urban males shows that the rate is very low up to 30 years. It increases rapidly until the maximum is reached at age 40 to 44 years. The rate then remains nearly stationary until age 60, when it undergoes a marked decline. The general average rates in this clinical group are: Urban males, 8.5; rural males, 2.5; urban females, 1.1; rural females, 0.1.

Chart 6 is based on 14,031 dementia præcox first admissions. This group is of special interest because it greatly outnumbers any other single clinical group. The group also has tremendous economic significance, as the onset of the disorder occurs comparatively early in life. The curves shown in Chart 6 correspond quite closely to similar curves worked out for over 9,000 cases in New York State. It is believed that the chart forms a fairly good picture of the variations in rates of the admissions of the two sexes from urban and rural environments. It is apparent from the chart that the rate in cities is very much higher than in rural districts. The rate among urban males is especially high in the early age groups. It shoots up rapidly from age 20 and reaches its maximum during the age period 25 to 29 years. During the succeeding quinquennial period it declines slightly and in the following periods the decline is very rapid. The rate for rural males is much lower than that for urban males but the maximum rate is reached at the same age period. The rate for urban females is much lower than that for urban males in the age groups under 35 to 39 years and much higher in the groups beyond that age. The maximum rate for both urban and rural females is reached in the age group 30 to 34 years. The rate for rural females is the lowest of all. The general average rates in this clinical group are: Urban males, 27.9; urban females, 21.6; rural males, 14.9; rural females, 11.7.

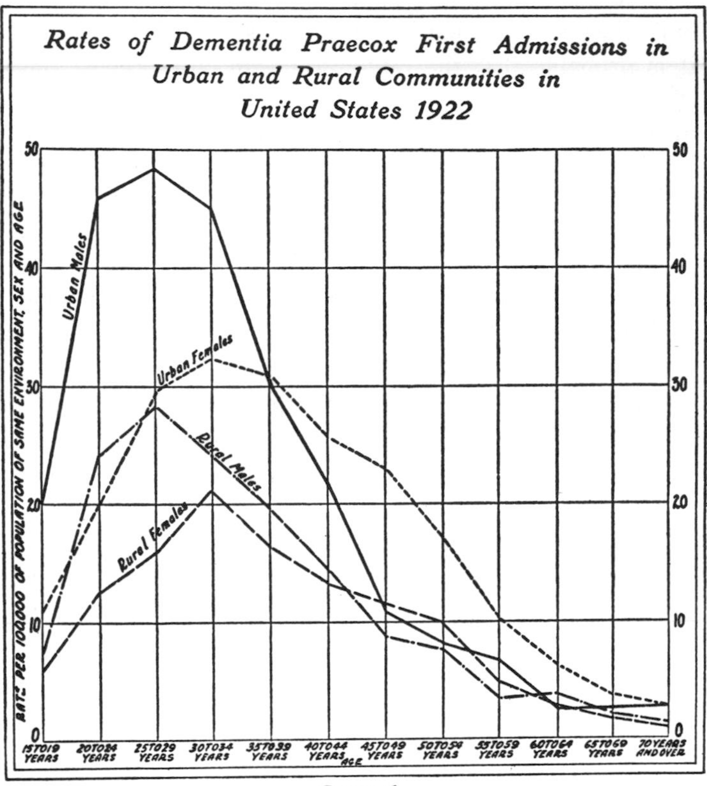

CHART 6.

Chart 7 is based on 10,028 manic-depressive first admissions. In this clinical group the rates for females greatly exceed those for males, the most marked differences being in the middle period of life. The highest rate is found among urban females, the curve for this group being fairly symmetrical and reaching its maximum in the age period 45 to 49 years. The curve for rural females falls below that for urban females and reaches its maximum about five years earlier. The curve for rural males reaches its peak at age period 50 to 54 years and that for urban males in age period 55 to 59 years. It will be noted that there is marked correlation between the two curves for females and also between the two curves for males indicating that sex is an important factor in this mental disorder. The general average rates for the four groups are: Urban females, 18.2; rural females, 14.6; urban males, 11.8; rural males, 11.2.

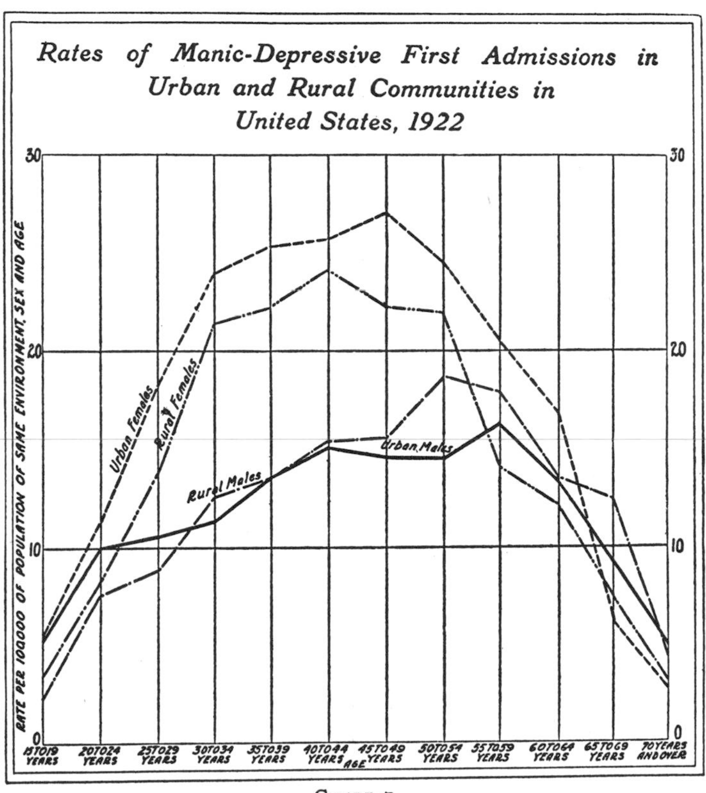

CHART 7.

Chart 8 has to do with 1,556 first admissions with involution melancholia. As would be expected the curves in this chart bear some resemblance to those in the chart relating to manic-depressive admissions, but the rates are much lower and the age groups repsented are more advanced. Urban females have the highest rate in this group at all periods of life. The rate for rural females is higher than the rates for urban and rural males during the early life periods, but in the age group 55 to 59 years, the rate for urban males exceeds that for rural females. Rural males are represented by very low rates in this group. The general average rates in this clinical group are: Urban females, 9.6; rural females, 5.9; urban males, 4.1; rural males, 2.5.

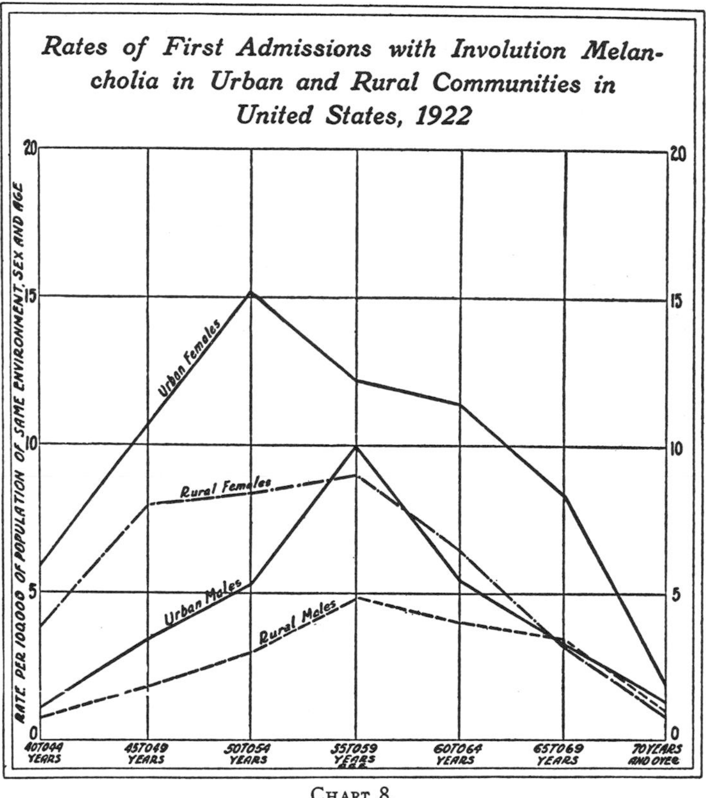

CHART 8.

Chart 9 deals with 2,538 first admissions with psychoneuroses and neuroses. The most striking feature of this chart is the high rates for urban males in the age periods between 20 and 35 years. The rural males also have their highest rates during the same age periods, but the rates are very much less than those of urban males. A considerable part of these male cases are ex-service men. The general average rates in this group are: Urban males, 5.6; urban females, 3.5; rural males, 2.6; rural females, 2.0.

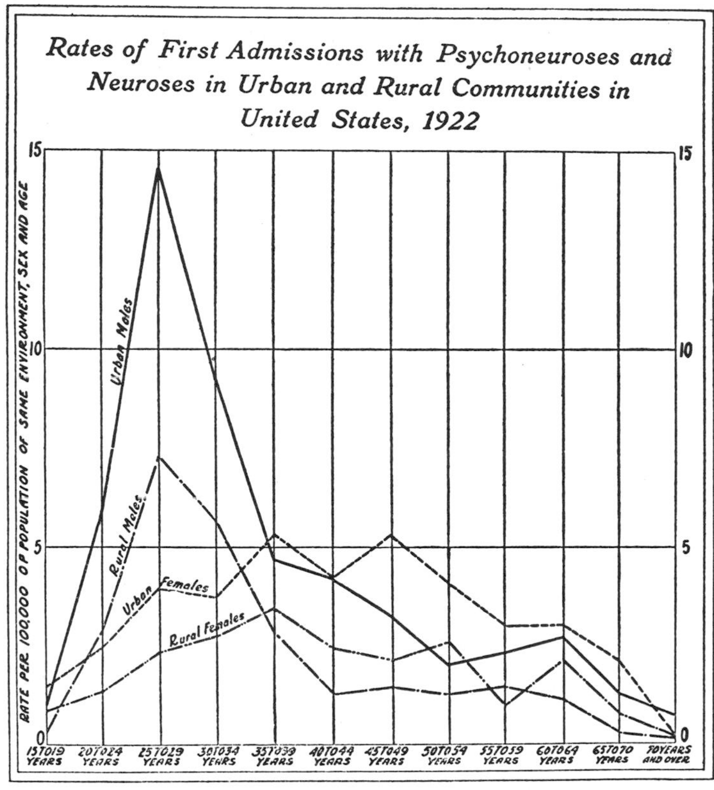

Chart 9

The causes of the variations in rates that have been pointed out in these charts are but partly known. To discuss them adequately would take us far beyond the limits of this paper. The variations have great significance and should be taken into account by anyone attempting preventive work. Mental disease in the future will be largely a city problem. Syphilis and alcoholism can and should be eradicated. But aside from these it appears that the complexities of our large cities require more adjustments than many individuals are equipped to make. To better the situation it will be necessary to strengthen the individual and to lessen the stresses of city life. To accomplish this task will require the united efforts of parents, teachers, physicians and social and research workers on the one hand; and of employers, industrial leaders, city managers and economists on the other.

CHAPTER X

The Future of Mental Disease from a Statistical Viewpoint*

Forecasting the future has always been a favorite diversion. People of all ages have taken deep interest in what the future had in store for them. The oracles, prophets and magicians of ancient times who could guess successfully concerning future events did a thriving business and won great renown, but if they guessed wrongly they lost their jobs and sometimes their heads. The survivors, therefore, got into the habit of giving their prophecies in mysterious and ambiguous language, so that they were able to justify themselves regardless of the course of events. This acquired characteristic seems to have been inherited by their modern successors, the fortune-tellers, clairvoyants, meteorologists and statisticians. Notwithstanding such precautions, none of the latter has made a complete success of the business of peering into the future, although all have found it more or less profitable. So long as human nature remains what it is, the fortune-teller will be in demand, and the religious enthusiast that can foretell with absolute assurance the fate of the world will have many followers. The weather prophet and the statistical forecaster, who have reduced their business to a science, are also in great demand. One well known statistical organization is employing more than 300 persons in its business of telling fortune-hunters what to expect in the stock market. Several government and state offices are now busily engaged in estimating future crops and business conditions for the benefit of the public, and only last month the distinguished head of the New York State Department of Health employed statistics to foretell the probable increase in average longevity during the next 20 years.

With these precedents I feel justified in telling you what statistics have to say concerning the business in which you are engaged. At the outset I wish to allay any apprehensions you may have concerning the permanence of your positions. Unless the theory of probability fails and statistical curves are meaningless, the hospitals for the treatment of mental disease will be among the last institutions to go out of business when this old world "has run its

*Read at annual meeting of American Psychiatric Association at Detroit, June 22, 1923.

course and the heavens are rolled up like a scroll," and judging from present conditions, there will be vacancies on the medical staffs up to the very last.

The institutions for mental disease in this country have expanded marvelously since 1880. The facts as set forth by various census reports are shown in the accompanying table.

TABLE 1. PATIENTS WITH MENTAL DISEASE IN INSTITUTIONS, 1880-1920

Year	Number	Per 100,000 of general population
1880	40,942	81.6
1890	74,028	118.2
1904	150,151	183.6
1910	187,791	204.2
1918	223,957	217.5
1920	232,680	220.1

We do not infer from this table that the rate of incidence of mental disease has increased so enormously, but that a constantly increasing proportion of mental patients is being cared for in institutions. The proportion of the population suffering from mental disease also seems to have increased. There has been a growing confidence on the part of the public in institutions for the treatment of mental patients, and as the death rate among such patients is probably much less in institutions than in homes, there has been a steady accumulation of patients, although the rate of incidence of mental disease has not so markedly increased. (See Chart 1.)

The accompanying chart (No. 1) tells its own story. The experience of New York State is similar to that of the whole country, but as State care in New York has a longer history than in most states, the accumulation of patients is relatively greater.

Many influences for and against mental health are seen in our modern civilization. An analysis of some of these will help in forecasting the future.

The most striking phenomenon in this connection may be stated as a paradoxical principle, namely: *Mental disease increases as physical disease decreases.* The truth of this principle may be demonstrated by elaborate tables, but a simple illustration will suffice. Suppose, for example, that some physical disease became so preva-

CHART 1

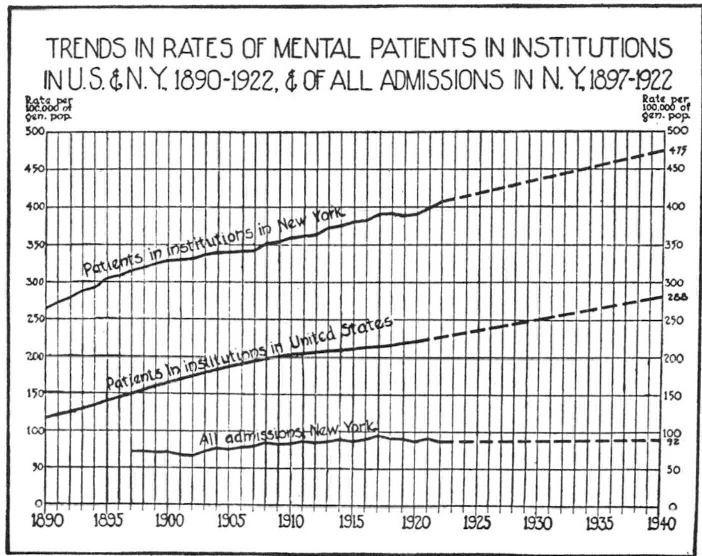

lent and so fatal that most people succumbed to it before reaching the age of 25. Mental disease would then greatly decline, as comparatively few persons develop mental disorders before reaching that age. On the other hand, suppose that infectious diseases and the diseases of early life were all eradicated and the average longevity reached 70 years or more, mental disease would then enormously increase as the rate of incidence of mental disease mounts up with advancing age. (See Chart 2.)

This paradoxical principle has been operating during the past 40 years, while the average length of life in the United States has advanced from about 41 to 56 years. We have every reason to believe that the principle will continue to operate as more physical diseases are conquered.

A second principle steadily working to furnish more patients for your institutions is this: *The rate of mental disease is higher in cities than in rural districts.* This principle, I believe, has always been true, in spite of the widely circulated legend to the contrary. There is a prevalent tradition that the rate of mental disease is

CHART 2

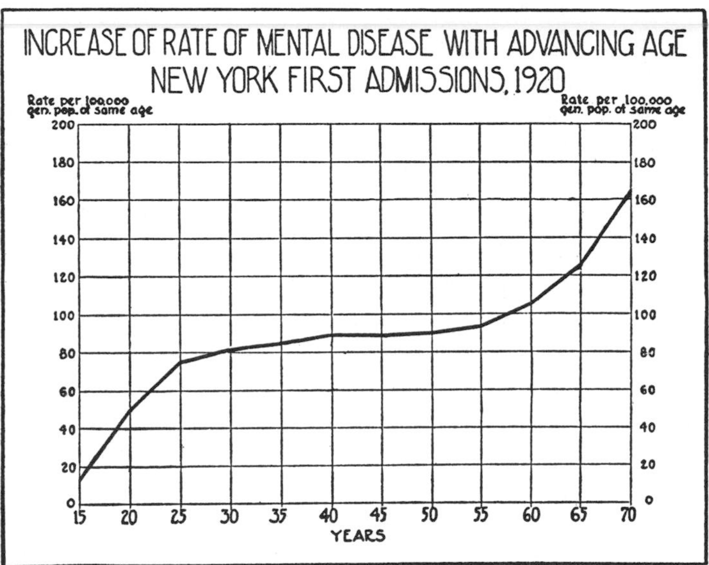

extremely high among farmers' wives. I have sought in vain for the origin of that tradition and for its basis in fact. We now know that farmers' wives are conspicuously free from mental disease, more so even than farmers, and farmers have much less mental disease than their city brothers. (See Table 2.)

The shifting of the population of the United States from rural to urban, that has been going on since 1880, is seen in the accompanying table. (No. 3.)

Our cities are still rapidly growing and our rural population is relatively declining. We may therefore expect further increases from this cause in the rate of mental disease from the population as a whole. (See Table 3.)

A third principle which is operating to increase mental disease has to do with eugenics. It may be roughly stated in these words: *The rate of mental disease is higher among inferior stocks than among superior stocks.* There are many facts that might be cited in support of this principle, but as the Census Bureau takes no account of the quality of family stock, the operation of the principle in the whole country cannot be demonstrated. The general birth-rate in late years has markedly declined, and it is generally believed that the decline has been greatest among superior stocks. If this trend continues, future peoples will become more and more susceptible to mental disease.

TABLE 2. RATES OF MENTAL DISEASE IN URBAN AND RURAL DISTRICTS IN NEW YORK STATE, 1915-1920

Psychoses	Urban first admissions		Rural first admissions	
	Number	Average Annual rate per 100,000	Number	Average Annual rate per 100,000
Senile	2,535	6.2	596	6.4
Cerebral arteriosclerosis	1,698	4.2	332	3.5
General paralysis	3,987	9.8	267	2.9
Cerebral syphilis	186	0.5	24	0.3
Alcoholic	1,510	3.7	152	1.6
With other somatic diseases	839	2.1	125	1.3
Manic depressive	3,839	9.4	570	6.1
Involution melancholia	855	2.1	275	2.9
Dementia præcox	7,790	19.1	728	7.8
Paranoia or paranoic conditions	535	1.3	94	1.0
Epileptic	652	1.6	106	1.1
With psychopathic personality	558	1.4	110	1.2
With mental deficiency	702	1.7	202	2.2
All other psychoses	2,696	6.6	392	4.2
Total	28,382	69.5	3,973	42.5

PER CENT DISTRIBUTION OF URBAN AND RURAL POPULATION IN UNITED STATES, 1880-1920

Year	Urban	Rural
1880	28.6	71.4
1890	35.4	64.6
1900	40.0	60.0
1910	45.8	54.2
1920	51.4	48.6

If there were no factors tending to counteract these influences, the prospect would be dark indeed. Many forces, however, are working to check the flowing tide of mental disease, and their effects are already being felt. The factor most widely discussed at the present time is the prohibition of the liquor traffic. Although the extent of the influence of alcohol as a cause of mental disease has at times been grossly exaggerated, the passing of the traffic would eliminate one of the principal groups of psychoses and will tend to reduce admissions in other groups. (See Chart 3.)

The movement to check the spread of syphilis, which acquired considerable impetus during the war and has since been continued, has great significance in the field of mental health. Syphilis for many years has been the primary cause of the mental disorder of more than one-eighth of the first admissions to the institutions for mental disease in New York State, and of a somewhat less proportion in the country as a whole. Syphilis can and will be brought under control. When this is accomplished another of the large groups of psychoses will disappear. (See Chart 3.)

Chart 3

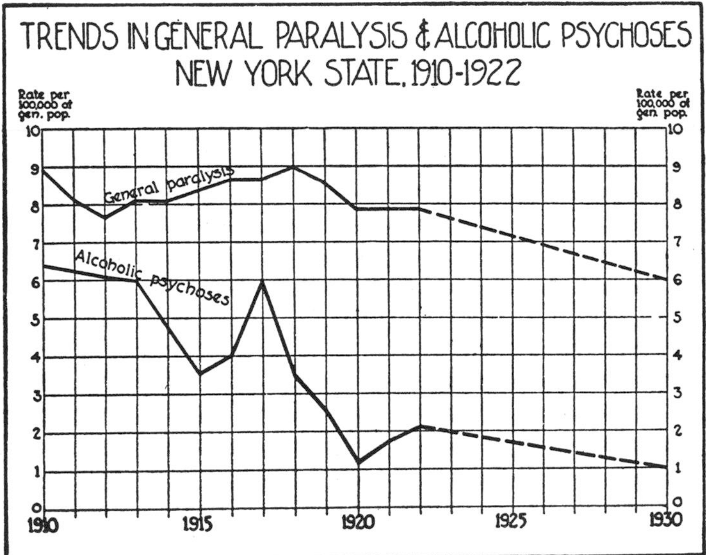

Many factors are operating to reduce mental disease, but their general results are not easily measured. They include psychopathic hospitals, mental clinics, psychiatric social work, and mental hygiene measures of various kinds. Much of the work being done in this field is experimental, but on the whole it is very promising.

To forecast the future after taking into account the various forces working for and against mental health is a difficult matter. We know what has happened in recent years and we know present conditions. From these we can determine trends which may be projected into the future. This has been done in the accompanying charts. These indicate a continually increasing rate of mental patients in institutions and a nearly stationary incidence rate of mental disease as shown by admissions. (Chart 1.) Alcoholic first admissions showed a marked decline from 1910 to 1923, and general paralysis first admissions a slight decline since 1918. (Chart 3.) The rates of dementia præcox and manic-depressive psychoses are both increasing. (Chart 4.)

CHART 4

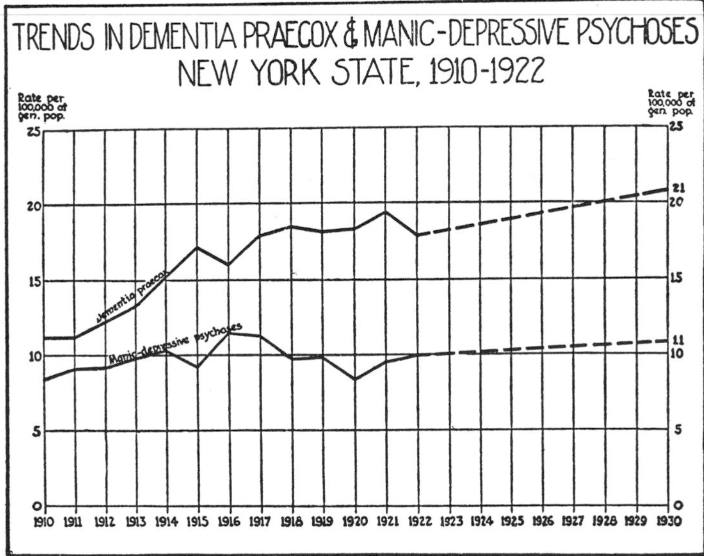

The rate of senile psychoses remains nearly stationary, while that of psychoses with cerebral arteriosclerosis is notably increasing. (Chart 5.) The smaller groups of psychoses are not shown in the charts, as individually they have little significance in determining the general trend.

CHART 5

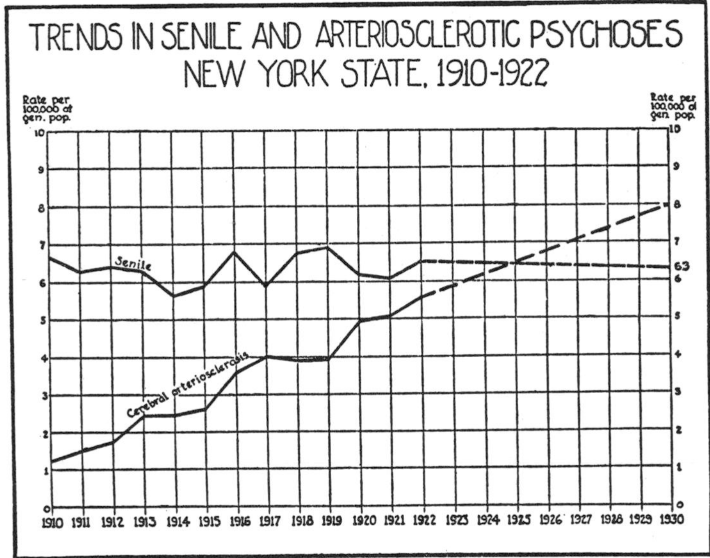

Much has been learned concerning the causes and nature of the various abnormal mental conditions, but comparatively little concerning curative treatment and prevention. Our present knowledge of mental diseases may be likened to the knowledge of infectious diseases of 1880. If some great research worker like Pasteur should come and tell us how to prevent dementia præcox and manic-depressive psychoses the whole aspect of the problem would be changed. It is not unlikely that important discoveries in this field will soon be made, but if they are not made, we may, in the not distant future, expect that mental disease will supersede physical disease as the paramount health problem.

Although the immediate outlook for mental health from the stand point of society is somewhat depressing, it is not without hope. We can take courage from what has been accomplished in the field of physical disease, and we may confidently expect that by multiplying means of research and by diligently disseminating the recently acquired knowledge of mental hygiene, the burden of mental disease will be lessened for future generations.

CHAPTER XI

WHAT HAPPENS TO PATIENTS WITH MENTAL DISEASE DURING THE FIRST YEAR OF HOSPITAL LIFE*

It has long been observed that the first year of hospital life is the most critical period in the life history of most patients with mental disease, but ordinary hospital statistics throw little light on the matter.

In order to find out more definitely what happens to the patients of the several clinical groups in the civil State hospitals of New York during their first hospital year, a study of 200 consecutive first admissions of each principal group was undertaken. To eliminate the influence of the late war and to cover a period when the medical and nursing personnel of the hospitals was on a satisfactory basis, the first admissions of a period beginning October 1, 1914, were selected. Altogether the study covered 16 psychotic groups comprising a total of 3,200 patients. The following small groups were not included: Traumatic psychoses, psychoses with Huntington's chorea, psychoses with brain tumor, psychoses due to drugs and other exogenous toxins and psychoses with pellagra. The data derived from the statistical cards of each group studied were tabulated separately, and from these separate tabulations, were prepared percentage tables comparing results in the 16 groups.

The term "hospital year," as used in this study, refers not to a fiscal or calendar year, but to a full year from the date of admission of each patient unless death or discharge earlier occurred.

The term "recovered" denotes the condition of a patient who has regained his normal health so that he may be considered as having practically the same mental status as he had previous to the onset of his psychosis.

The term "improved" includes also the "much improved" and denotes any degree of mental gain less than *recovered* which warrants the patient's discharge.

The term "unimproved" denotes no mental gain, and applies to patients discharged for removal to their homes in other states or countries, or to the care of relatives.

*Published in State Hospital Quarterly, August, 1925.

Senile Psychoses

Of the 200 senile first admissions, 125 died during the first year of hospital life. That many of these were acutely ill at the time of admission is shown by the fact that 44 died within one month after admission and 34 additional in the next two months. Only 11 of the 200 cases were discharged as improved during the year; 52 remained under treatment at the end of their first year.

Table 1. Results During First Year of Hospital Life
200 consecutive first admissions with senile psychoses

	Time after admission								
	Total	Under 1 mo.	1-2 mos.	3-4 mos.	5-6 mos.	7-8 mos.	9-10 mos.	11-12 mos.	Readm. within year
Discharged:									
Recovered	..	..	..	..	..	..	..	..	..
Improved	11	..	2	1	4	2	1	1	..
Unimproved	12	4	4	2	..	1	..	1	..
Died	125	44	34	12	10	10	8	7	..
Remaining in hospital:									
Not discharged	52	..	..	..	..	..	..	..	..
Readmitted	..	..	..	..	..	..	..	..	..

Psychoses with Cerebral Arteriosclerosis

Of the 200 first admissions of the group of psychoses with cerebral arteriosclerosis, 10 were discharged as recovered and 25 as improved during the first year of hospital life. Ninety-seven patients

Table 2. Results During First Year of Hospital Life
200 consecutive first admissions with psychoses with cerebral arteriosclerosis

	Time after admission								
	Total	Under 1 mo.	1-2 mos.	3-4 mos.	5-6 mos.	7-8 mos.	9-10 mos.	11-12 mos.	Readm. within year
Discharged:									
Recovered	10	..	3	2	3	2	..	..	..
Improved	25	3	10	8	1	2	..	1	..
Unimproved	11	5	2	2	2	..	..	..	3
Died	97	20	28	19	9	8	9	4	..
Remaining in hospital:									
Not discharged	54	..	..	..	..	..	..	..	..
Readmitted	3	..	..	..	..	..	..	..	..

died in the hospital. Of these, 20 died within one month after admission and 28 additional in the two succeeding months. Three discharged cases were subsequently readmitted. A total of 57 cases remained under treatment beyond the first year.

General Paralysis

The proportion of deaths in the general paresis group during the first hospital year was less than in the senile and cerebral arteriosclerotic groups, the numbers being 90, 125 and 97, respectively. No recoveries occurred, but 17 cases were discharged as improved. Two of these cases were subsequently readmitted. Of the 90 deaths, 18 occurred within one month of admission, 19 in the period one to two months, 21 in the period three to four months, and 12 in the period five to six months. Seventy-nine of the 200 cases remained under treatment at the end of their hospital year.

TABLE 3. RESULTS DURING FIRST YEAR OF HOSPITAL LIFE
200 consecutive first admissions with general paresis

	Time after admission								
	Total	Under 1 mo.	1-2 mos.	3-4 mos.	5-6 mos.	7-8 mos.	9-10 mos.	11-12 mos.	Readm. within year
Discharged:									
Recovered	..	..	..	..	..	..	..	..	..
Improved	17	1	5	2	6	1	2	..	2
Unimproved	14	4	4	4	1	1	..	..	1
Died	90	18	19*	21	12	7	5	8	..
Remaining in hospital:									
Not discharged	77	..	..	..	..	..	..	..	..
Readmitted	2	..	..	..	..	..	..	..	..

*Includes one readmission.

Psychoses with Cerebral Syphilis

Results in the group of psychoses with cerebral syphilis during the first year of hospital life are much more favorable than in the general paresis group. Of the 200 first admissions, 15 were discharged as recovered and 34 as improved. Of the 75 patients that died, 48 were in the hospital less than five months. Of the discharged cases two were readmitted during the year. These and 63 others remained under treatment at the end of the first year.

TABLE 4. RESULTS DURING FIRST YEAR OF HOSPITAL LIFE
200 consecutive first admissions with psychoses with cerebral syphilis

	Time after admission								
	Total	Under 1 mo.	1-2 mos.	3-4 mos.	5-6 mos.	7-8 mos.	9-10 mos.	11-12 mos.	Readm. within year
Discharged:									
Recovered	15	2	1	5	3	..	3	1	..
Improved	34	2	11	11	3	2	3	2	1
Unimproved	11	5	3	2	..	1	..	..	1
Died	75	23	14	11	7	13	4	3	..
Remaining in hospital:									
Not discharged	63	..	..	..	..	..	..	..	..
Readmitted	2	..	..	..	..	..	..	..	..

PSYCHOSES WITH OTHER BRAIN OR NERVOUS DISEASES

Results in this composite organic group appear more favorable than would be expected. Of the 200 first admissions, 29 were discharged as recovered and 29 others as improved. Sixty-nine of the patients died, death occurring within one month in 35 cases, and within five months in 26 additional cases; 64 cases remained under treatment at the end of the hospital year.

TABLE 5. RESULTS DURING FIRST YEAR OF HOSPITAL LIFE
200 consecutive first admissions with psychoses with other brain or nervous diseases

	Time after admission								
	Total	Under 1 mo.	1-2 mos.	3-4 mos.	5-6 mos.	7-8 mos.	9-10 mos.	11-12 mos.	Readm. within year
Discharged:									
Recovered	29	3	11	5	3	2	2	3	..
Improved	29	3	7	11	3	2	3	..	..
Unimproved	9	1	3	1	2	2	..	..	..
Died	69	35	13	13	1	5	2	..	..
Remaining in hospital:									
Not discharged	64	..	..	..	..	..	..	..	..
Readmitted	..	..	..	..	..	..	..	..	..

ALCOHOLIC PSYCHOSES

Patients with alcoholic psychoses constitute in the main a benign group. Of the 200 first admissions studied, 102 were discharged as recovered within a year from admission; of these, 94 were discharged during the first six months of hospital life; 24 cases were discharged as improved and only 12 of the 200 cases died in the hospital. Fifty-four remained under treatment at the end of the hospital year.

TABLE 6. RESULTS DURING FIRST YEAR OF HOSPITAL LIFE
200 consecutive first admissions with alcoholic psychoses

	Time after admission								
	Total	Under 1 mo.	1-2 mos.	3-4 mos.	5-6 mos.	7-8 mos.	9-10 mos.	11-12 mos.	Readm. within year
Discharged:									
Recovered	102	20	34*	30*	10*	2	5	1	2
Improved	24	4	10	4	4	2	..	..	1
Unimproved	8	2	2*	2	1	..	1	..	1
Died	12	6	..	2	1	1	2	..	..
Remaining in hospital:									
Not discharged	54	..	..	..	..	..	..	..	..
Readmitted	..	..	..	..	..	..	..	..	..

*Includes one readmission.

PSYCHOSES WITH OTHER SOMATIC DISEASES

This composite group includes many cases who are acutely ill at the time of admission. This is indicated by the fact that 68 of the 200 patients died during the first month of hospital life, and 21 more during the subsequent two months. The results shown in the accompanying table indicate that in a large percentage of cases in this group recovery may be expected if the physical disease is overcome.

TABLE 7. RESULTS DURING FIRST YEAR OF HOSPITAL LIFE
200 consecutive first admissions with psychoses with other somatic diseases

	Time after admission								
	Total	Under 1 mo.	1-2 mos.	3-4 mos.	5-6 mos.	7-8 mos.	9-10 mos.	11-12 mos.	Readm. within year
Discharged:									
Recovered	70	12	30	21	3	2	2	..	..
Improved	14	6	7	1	..	..	..	..	..
Unimproved	5	2	2	1	..	..	..	..	..
Died	97	68	21	3	4	1	..	..	..
Remaining in hospital:									
Not discharged	14	..	..	..	..	..	..	..	..
Readmitted	..	..	..	..	..	..	..	..	..

Manic-Depressive Psychoses

Of the 200 manic-depressive cases studied, exactly 100 were discharged as recovered during the first hospital year. Of these, 51 were under treatment less than seven months and 49 from seven to twelve months. Thirty-five additional patients were discharged as improved. Five of the discharged cases were readmitted, and at the end of the first year of treatment 41 remained in the hospital.

Table 8. Results During First Year of Hospital Life
200 consecutive first admissions with manic-depressive psychoses

	Time after admission								
	Total	Under 1 mo.	1-2 mos.	3-4 mos.	5-6 mos.	7-8 mos.	9-10 mos.	11-12 mos.	Readm. within year
Discharged:									
Recovered	100	5	9	15	22*	31*	13	5	3
Improved	35	5	7	3	6	7*	3	4*	2
Unimproved	4	2	..	2	..	..	..	..	..
Died	20	11	1	..	2	3	3	..	..
Remaining in hospital:									
Not discharged	40	..	..	..	..	..	..	..	..
Readmitted	1	..	..	..	..	..	..	..	..

*Includes one readmission.

Involution Melancholia

While the reactions of the involution group are similar to those of the manic-depressive group, the patients are much older and consequently the results obtained from hospital treatment are less

Table 9. Results During First Year of Hospital Life
200 consecutive first admissions with involution melancholia

	Time after admission								
	Total	Under 1 mo.	1-2 mos.	3-4 mos.	5-6 mos.	7-8 mos.	9-10 mos.	11-12 mos.	Readm. within year
Discharged:									
Recovered	31	..	5	12	5	2	3	4	..
Improved	25	6	5	2	5	3	2	2	1
Unimproved	12	5	4	1	2	..	..	..	2
Died	45	13	11*	9	4	2	3	3	..
Remaining in hospital:									
Not discharged	85	..	..	..	..	..	..	..	..
Readmitted	2	..	..	..	..	..	..	..	..

*Includes one readmission.

favorable. Of the 200 involution melancholia cases studied, only 31 were discharged as recovered during their first hospital year; 25 others were discharged as improved, and 45 died in the hospital. Twenty-four of these died before having been in the hospital three months. Three of the discharged cases were readmitted, and 87 remained under treatment at the end of their hospital year.

Dementia Præcox

The prolonged course of dementia præcox is clearly indicated by the results shown in the accompanying table. Of the 200 cases studied, only 3 were discharged as recovered during their first hospital year, 42 were discharged as improved and 3 died in the hospital. One of the patients discharged as recovered and 2 of those discharged as improved were readmitted. One hundred thirty-three patients remained under treatment at the end of their first hospital year.

Table 10. Results During First Year of Hospital Life
200 consecutive first admissions with dementia præcox

	Total	Time after admission							
		Under 1 mo.	1-2 mos.	3-4 mos.	5-6 mos.	7-8 mos.	9-10 mos.	11-12 mos.	Readm. within year
Discharged:									
Recovered	3	..	2	..	1	..	..	..	1
Improved	42	4	6	10	8	7	4	3	2
Unimproved	19	6	10	1	1	..	1	..	..
Died	3	..	1	..	..	1	1*	..	..
Remaining in hospital:									
Not discharged	131	..	..	..	..	..	..	..	..
Readmitted	2	..	..	..	..	..	..	..	..

*Includes one readmission.

Paranoia or Paranoid Conditions

The most striking results shown in the tabulation of the paranoid cases is the large number of cases discharged as improved, there being 61 of these, while only 12 were discharged as recovered. Thirteen of the patients died, 5 of the discharged cases were readmitted and 92 remained in the hospital after one year of treatment.

TABLE 11. RESULTS DURING FIRST YEAR OF HOSPITAL LIFE

200 consecutive first admissions with paranoia or paranoid conditions

	Time after admission								
	Total	Under 1 mo.	1-2 mos.	3-4 mos.	5-6 mos.	7-8 mos.	9-10 mos.	11-12 mos.	Readm. within year
Discharged:									
Recovered	12	..	5	3	..	2	1	1	1
Improved	61	9	17	17*	11	5	2	..	2
Unimproved	22	4	6	2	5	..	4	1*	2
Died	13	2	..	8	1	..	1	1	..
Remaining in hospital:									
Not discharged	89	..	..	..	..	..	..	..	..
Readmitted	3	..	..	..	..	..	..	..	..

*Includes one readmission.

EPILEPTIC PSYCHOSES

Results in the epileptic group are more favorable than would be expected. Thirty-two of the 200 cases were discharged as having recovered from their psychotic episode within the first hospital year; 18 of these were discharged within less than three months after admission. Twenty additional cases were discharged as improved; 7 of the discharged cases were readmitted during the year; 16 of the patients died, and 123 remained in the hospital at the close of their year of treatment.

TABLE 12. RESULTS DURING FIRST YEAR OF HOSPITAL LIFE

200 consecutive first admissions with epileptic psychoses

	Time after admission								
	Total	Under 1 mo.	1-2 mos.	3-4 mos.	5-6 mos.	7-8 mos.	9-10 mos.	11-12 mos.	Readm. within year
Discharged:									
Recovered	32	2	16	7*	3	4	..	..	4
Improved	20	4	7*	3	5	..	..	1*	1
Unimproved	9	6	..	..	1	2	..	..	2
Died	16	..	1	4	5*	2	2	2	..
Remaining in hospital:									
Not discharged	120	..	..	..	..	..	..	..	..
Readmitted	3	..	..	..	..	..	..	..	..

*Includes one readmission.

Psychoneuroses and Neuroses

Highly beneficial results are secured in the treatment of patients with psychoneuroses and neuroses. Out of the 200 first admissions tabulated, 63 were discharged as recovered within their first hospital year and 73 additional were discharged as improved; only 5 of the patients died in the hospital; 4 of the discharged cases were readmitted and 41 continued in the hospital. It is noteworthy that the proportion of total cases discharged as recovered and improved in this group exceeds that of any other group.

Table 13. Results During First Year of Hospital Life
200 consecutive first admissions with psychoneuroses and neuroses

	Time after admission								
	Total	Under 1 mo.	1-2 mos.	3-4 mos.	5-6 mos.	7-8 mos.	9-10 mos.	11-12 mos.	Readm. within year
Discharged:									
Recovered	63	8	27	14*	6	2	5	1	3
Improved	73	21*	23	9*	9	6	3	2	1
Unimproved	18	11	1	1	2	2	1	..	..
Died	5	..	4	..	1	..	..	..	..
Remaining in hospital:									
Not discharged	40	..	..	..	..	..	..	..	..
Readmitted	1	..	..	..	..	..	..	..	..

*Includes one readmission.

Table 14. Results During First Year of Hospital Life
200 consecutive first admissions with psychoses with psychopathic personality

	Time after admission								
	Total	Under 1 mo.	1-2 mos.	3-4 mos.	5-6 mos.	7-8 mos.	9-10 mos.	11-12 mos.	Readm. within year
Discharged:									
Recovered	82	8	17	22**	25†	4	3	3	5
Improved	42	4*	11	15	4	3	2	3	1
Unimproved	10	3	5	2	..	..	..	..	3
Died	4	2	1	..	..	1	..	..	..
Remaining in hospital:									
Not discharged	59	..	..	..	..	..	..	..	..
Readmitted	3	..	..	..	..	..	..	..	..

*Includes one readmission.
**Includes two readmissions.
†Includes three readmissions.

Psychoses with Psychopathic Personality

Gratifying results also appear in the data concerning the group psychoses with psychopathic personality. Eighty-two of the 200 first admissions studied were discharged as recovered and 42 as improved during the first hospital year. Of the 82 recovered cases, 72 were in the hospital less than seven months. Only 4 patients died in the hospital. Nine of the discharged cases were readmitted during the year and 62 continued under treatment.

Psychoses with Mental Deficiency

Of the 200 first admissions in the group, psychoses with mental deficiency, 60 were discharged as having recovered from their psychotic episode during their first hospital year and 26 additional as being improved. Of the 60 cases discharged as recovered, 48 were in the hospital less than seven months. Thirteen of the patients died, 4 of the discharged cases were readmitted and 95 remained under treatment at the end of their first hospital year.

Table 15. Results During First Year of Hospital Life

200 consecutive first admissions with psychoses with mental deficiency

	Time after admission								
	Total	Under 1 mo.	1-2 mos.	3-4 mos.	5-6 mos.	7-8 mos.	9-10 mos.	11-12 mos.	Readm. within year
Discharged:									
Recovered	60	4	14*	13	17	5	5*	2	2
Improved	26	1	11	3	7	3	..	1	2
Unimproved	6	1	1	2	2	..	..	..	..
Died	13	4	3	..	2	2	1	1	..
Remaining in hospital:									
Not discharged	93	..	..	..	..	..	..	..	..
Readmitted	2	..	..	..	..	..	..	..	..

*Includes one readmission.

Undiagnosed Psychoses

The undiagnosed group consists of cases that cannot be readily classified. The difficulty in placing them in one of the definite groups may be due to unusual symptoms, lack of information or to death during the period of observation. Of the 200 cases in this group, 47 were discharged as recovered and 31 as improved; 48 died in the hospital. In 40 of these cases death occurred within two months of the time of admission; 52 continued under treatment at the end of their first hospital year.

TABLE 16. RESULTS DURING FIRST YEAR OF HOSPITAL LIFE

200 consecutive first admissions with undiagnosed psychoses

	Time after admission								
	Total	Under 1 mo.	1-2 mos.	3-4 mos.	5-6 mos.	7-8 mos.	9-10 mos.	11-12 mos.	Readm. within year
Discharged:									
Recovered	47	8	15	13	4	2	3	2	..
Improved	31	6	9	7	5	4	..	..	..
Unimproved	22	10	6	2	2	1	1	..	..
Died	48	28	12	4	1	..	3	..	..
Remaining in hospital:									
Not discharged	52	..	..	..	..	..	..	..	..
Readmitted	..	..	..	..	..	..	..	..	..

COMPARATIVE SUMMARY

Table 17 gives a comparative summary of the departures from the hospital at specified periods. Of the entire group of 3,200 patients, 65.3 per cent were out of the hospital at the end of one year, and 34.7 per cent remained under treatment; 15.5 per cent left the hospital during the first month and 17.3 per cent during the next two months. A decreasing percentage left the hospital in each succeeding two months of the year. The highest percentage of cases of any single group leaving the hospital during the year is found in the group psychoses with other somatic diseases, and the lowest in the dementia præcox group. High percentages leaving during the first month are found in the senile, somatic diseases and undiagnosed groups.

Table 18 gives classified results of the first year of hospital life without regard to subdivisions of time. Of the entire group of 3,200 patients, 20.5 per cent were discharged as recovered; 15.9 per cent as improved; 22.9 per cent died; 1.6 per cent were readmitted, and 34.7 per cent remained in the hospital. The highest percentages of deaths are found in the senile, cerebral arteriosclerosis,

TABLE 17. PERCENTAGE OF FIRST ADMISSIONS LEAVING HOSPITAL AT SPECIFIED PERIODS

Psychoses	Total out of hospital at end of one year	Time after admission							
		Under 1 mo.	1-2 mos.	3-4 mos.	5-6 mos.	7-8 mos.	9-10 mos.	11-12 mos.	Readmitted within year
Senile	74.0	24.0	20.0	7.5	7.0	6.5	4.5	4.5	...
Arteriosclerosis	71.5	14.0	21.5	15.5	7.5	6.0	4.5	2.5	1.5
General paresis	60.5	11.5	14.0	13.5	9.5	4.5	3.5	4.0	1.5
Cerebral syphilis	67.5	16.0	14.5	14.5	6.5	8.0	5.0	3.0	1.0
With other brain or nervous diseases	68.0	21.0	17.0	15.0	4.5	5.5	3.5	1.5	...
Alcoholic	73.0	16.0	23.0	19.0	8.0	2.5	4.0	0.5	2.0
With other somatic diseases	93.0	44.0	30.0	13.0	3.5	1.5	1.0	...	...
Manic-depressive	79.5	11.5	8.5	10.0	15.0	20.5	9.5	4.5	2.5
Involution melancholia	56.5	12.0	12.5	12.0	8.0	3.5	4.0	4.5	1.5
Dementia præcox	33.5	5.0	9.5	5.5	5.0	4.0	3.0	1.5	1.5
Paranoia or paranoid conditions	54.0	7.5	14.0	15.0	8.5	3.5	4.0	1.5	2.5
Epileptic psychoses	38.5	6.0	12.0	7.0	7.0	4.0	1.0	1.5	3.5
Psychoneuroses and neuroses	79.5	20.0	27.5	12.0	9.0	5.0	4.5	1.5	2.0
Psychopathic personality	69.0	8.5	17.0	19.5	14.5	4.0	2.5	3.0	4.5
Mental deficiency	52.5	5.0	14.5	9.0	14.0	5.0	3.0	2.0	2.0
Undiagnosed	74.0	26.0	21.0	13.0	6.0	3.5	3.5	1.0	...
Total	65.3	15.5	17.3	12.6	8.3	5.5	3.8	2.3	1.6

TABLE 18. SUMMARY OF RESULTS OF TREATMENT OF PATIENTS WITH MENTAL DISEASE DURING FIRST YEAR OF HOSPITAL LIFE

Psychoses	Per cent						
	Total	Discharged			Died	Remaining	Readmitted
		Recovered	Improved	Unimproved			
Senile	100.0	...	5.5	6.0	62.5	26.0	...
Arteriosclerosis	100.0	5.0	12.5	5.5	48.5	28.5	1.5
General paresis	100.0	...	8.5	7.0	45.0	39.5	1.5
Cerebral syphilis	100.0	7.5	17.0	5.5	37.5	32.5	1.0
With other brain or nervous diseases	100.0	14.5	14.5	4.5	34.5	32.0	...
Alcoholic	100.0	51.0	12.0	4.0	6.0	27.0	2.0
With other somatic diseases	100.0	35.0	7.0	2.5	48.5	7.0	...
Manic-depressive	100.0	50.0	17.5	2.0	10.0	20.5	2.5
Involution melancholia	100.0	15.5	12.5	6.0	22.5	43.5	1.5
Dementia præcox	100.0	1.5	21.0	9.5	1.5	66.5	1.5
Paranoia or paranoid conditions	100.0	6.0	30.5	11.0	6.5	46.0	2.5
Epileptic psychoses	100.0	16.0	10.0	4.5	8.0	61.5	3.5
Psychoneuroses and neuroses	100.0	31.5	36.5	9.0	2.5	20.5	2.0
Psychopathic personality	100.0	41.0	21.0	5.0	2.0	31.0	4.5
With mental deficiency	100.0	30.0	13.0	3.0	6.5	47.5	2.0
Undiagnosed	100.0	23.5	15.5	11.0	24.0	26.0	...
Total	100.0	20.5	15.9	6.0	22.9	34.7	1.6

general paresis and somatic disease groups. The highest percentages of recoveries are found in the alcoholic, manic-depressive and psychopathic personality groups. The highest percentages discharged as improved are found in the psychoneurotic and paranoid groups. The highest percentages remaining under treatment appear in the dementia præcox and epileptic groups.

CHAPTER XII

A Statistical Study of 1,140 Dementia Præcox Patients Treated with Metrazol*

Treatment of selected dementia præcox patients with metrazol was begun in some of the New York civil State hospitals in the fall of 1937. During the following year the treatment came into use in all but three of such hospitals. Various types of treatment were tried: In many cases metrazol alone was used; in some cases metrazol and camphor were tried; and in others, metrazol and insulin were combined. In the cases included in this study, either metrazol alone or metrazol with camphor was employed. No cases in which insulin was used previous to, or during the metrazol treatment are included.

The aim of this study is to ascertain as definitely as possible what happened to the patients who received metrazol treatment and the relative efficacy of metrazol and insulin.

In preparation for the study, the civil State hospitals were requested to fill out and send to the central office a standard statistical card report concerning each case treated with metrazol. Such report was forwarded in each instance about one month after the termination of treatment. After eliminating the cards showing previous treatment with insulin and predominately camphor cases, there remained 1,140 cards which were deemed satisfactory for tabulation. The distribution of these cases by hospitals and the reported results are shown by Table 1. It will be observed that 329 cases were treated at Brooklyn State Hospital, 275 at Rockland State Hospital and 121 at Creedmoor State Hospital. Together these comprise 63.6 per cent of all the cases constituting the study. It will also be noted that five hospitals each reported less than 10 treated cases. The other hospitals reported from 14 to 71 cases.

Of the 1,140 patients, 645 were males and 495 females. The sex distribution of treated cases varied widely in the several hospitals. Rockland treated 194 males and 81 females while Brooklyn treated 194 females and 135 males.

*Read before the Quarterly Conference of the Department of Mental Hygiene, at Albany, N. Y., March 18, 1939.

TABLE 1. OUTCOME OF METRAZOL TREATMENT OF DEMENTIA PRÆCOX PATIENTS IN NEW YORK CIVIL STATE HOSPITALS, 1938

State hospitals	Total			Recovered			Much improved			Improved			Unimproved			Died		
	M.	F.	T.	M.	F.	T.	M.	F.	T.	M.	F.	T.	M.	F.	T.	M.	F.	T.
Brooklyn	135	194	329	5	..	5	26	13	39	46	70	116	57	110	167	1	1	2
Buffalo	24	22	46	..	..	..	..	4	4	10	8	18	14	10	24	..	..	..
Central Islip	39	21	60	..	..	..	4	1	5	4	2	6	31	18	49	..	..	..
Creedmoor	81	40	121	..	..	..	..	..	..	10	3	13	71	37	108	..	..	..
Gowanda	43	28	71	1	1	2	9	8	17	17	6	23	16	12	28	..	1	1
Harlem Valley	..	2	2	..	..	..	..	..	..	..	..	..	..	2	2	..	..	..
Hudson River	33	32	65	..	..	..	1	1	2	5	3	8	27	28	55	..	..	..
Kings Park	35	20	55	..	..	..	..	..	..	1	..	1	32	19	51	2	1	3
Manhattan	13	15	28	1	1	2	5	5	10	2	3	5	5	6	11	..	..	..
Marcy	24	28	52	..	1	1	4	5	9	7	6	13	13	16	29	..	..	..
Pilgrim	2	1	3	..	..	..	..	..	..	..	..	..	2	1	3	..	..	..
Psychiatric Institute	11	3	14	4	2	6	3	..	3	1	..	1	3	1	4	..	..	..
Rockland	194	81	275	..	..	..	15	8	23	55	18	73	124	55	179	..	..	..
St. Lawrence	5	4	9	..	..	..	..	..	..	1	1	2	4	3	7	..	..	..
Utica	3	..	3	2	..	2	..	..	..	..	..	..	1	..	1	..	..	..
Willard	3	4	7	..	..	..	..	1	1	..	..	..	3	3	6	..	..	..
Total*	645	495	1140	13	5	18	67	46	113	159	120	279	403	321	724	3	3	6

*Includes cases treated by all State hospitals.

TABLE 2. COMPARISON OF RESULTS OF METRAZOL TREATMENT AND OF INSULIN TREATMENT WITH RESULTS PREVIOUSLY OBTAINED WITHOUT SPECIAL DRUG TREATMENT

State hospitals	Metrazol-treated patients					Insulin-treated patients					Control group					
	Recovered	Much improved	Improved	Unimproved	Died	Recovered	Much improved	Improved	Unimproved	Died	Recovered	Much improved	Improved	Unimproved	Still in hospital	Died
Brooklyn	1.5	11.9	35.3	50.8	0.6	25.4	25.4	27.1	21.5	0.6	5.6	16.9	8.5	2.3	56.5	10.2
Buffalo	..	8.7	39.1	52.2	..	7.5	38.8	31.3	22.4	..	9.0	17.9	4.5	3.0	62.7	3.0
Central Islip	..	8.3	10.0	81.7	..	6.6	31.6	15.8	43.4	2.6	..	15.8	7.9	2.6	71.1	2.6
Creedmoor	..	..	10.7	89.3	..	15.8	26.3	28.9	28.9	..	2.6	5.3	2.6	..	84.2	5.3
Gowanda	2.8	23.9	32.4	39.4	1.4	40.6	34.4	12.5	6.3	6.3	12.5	3.1	..	12.5	68.8	3.1
Hudson River	..	3.1	12.3	84.6	..	2.7	6.7	28.0	58.7	4.0	1.3	8.0	8.0	10.7	64.0	8.0
Kings Park	..	..	1.8	92.7	5.5	1.8	35.1	19.3	42.1	1.8	1.8	12.3	7.0	7.0	71.9	..
Manhattan	7.1	35.7	17.9	39.3	..	..	24.0	40.0	28.0	8.0	..	..	20.0	..	76.0	4.0
Marcy	1.9	17.3	25.0	55.8	..	4.0	44.0	20.0	28.0	4.0	..	32.0	4.0	4.0	60.0	..
Rockland	..	8.4	26.5	65.1	..	..	25.5	29.8	44.7	..	2.1	12.8	17.0	..	63.8	4.3
Total*	1.6	9.9	24.5	63.5	0.5	12.9	27.1	25.3	33.4	1.3	3.5	11.2	7.4	7.5	65.8	4.6

*Includes cases treated by all State hospitals.

Recovery and improvement rates among treated patients in the several hospitals were far from uniform. The Psychiatric Institute reported 6 recoveries among 14 patients treated, while Rockland State Hospital reported no recoveries among 275 patients and Brooklyn State Hospital, 5 recoveries among 329 patients.

In Table 2 is shown a comparison of results in certain hospitals among metrazol-treated cases, insulin-treated cases and control cases that received no special drug treatment.* Rates were not computed for the hospitals treating less than 25 cases. In every hospital shown in the table, better results were obtained with the use of insulin than with the use of metrazol. In fact, it does not appear that metrazol gives better results than were previously obtained without special drug treatment. This conclusion should not be construed as implying that metrazol is without value. In certain instances it seems to produce remarkable results.

Outcome According to Type of Dementia Præcox

Table 3 shows the distribution of treated cases by types of dementia præcox and gives the rates of outcome among patients of each type. As only 26 cases of the simple type were treated, the rates shown for this type have little significance. Rates of recovery and improvement for the hebephrenic, catatonic, and paranoid types are significant and clearly indicate that better results were obtained among patients of the catatonic and paranoid types than among those of the hebephrenic type. Among treated patients of the last named type, 69.1 per cent were reported as unimproved as compared with 60.8 per cent for the catatonic group and 61.5 per cent for the paranoid group. Among females in the hebephrenic group, the percentage unimproved was 76.8.

Table 4 compares results in the several types obtained by metrazol and insulin treatment. The rates for insulin cases are taken from Malzberg's paper, mentioned above. The data indicate clearly the superiority of insulin therapy in each of the several types of dementia præcox.

*The insulin cases and the control cases are those described in Malzberg's paper on "Outcome of Insulin Treatment of One Thousand Patients with Dementia Præcox." See Psychiatric Quarterly, Vol. 12, No. 3, July, 1938.

TABLE 3. OUTCOME OF METRAZOL TREATMENT ACCORDING TO TYPE OF DEMENTIA PRÆCOX

Types	Total			Recovered			Much improved			Improved			Unimproved			Died		
	M.	F.	T.	M.	F.	T.	M.	F.	T.	M.	F.	T.	M.	F.	T.	M.	F.	T.
							Number											
Simple	19	7	26	1	..	1	1	..	1	2	..	2	15	7	22	..	..	..
Hebephrenic	193	95	288	3	..	3	15	9	24	47	13	60	126	73	199	2	..	2
Catatonic	190	228	418	4	4	8	22	24	46	45	62	107	119	135	254	..	3	3
Paranoid	239	158	397	5	1	6	28	13	41	64	41	105	141	103	244	1	..	1
Others and unclassified	4	7	11	..	..	..	1	..	1	1	4	5	2	3	5	..	..	..
Total	645	495	1140	13	5	18	67	46	113	159	120	279	403	321	724	3	3	6
							Per Cent											
Simple	100.0	100.0	100.0	5.3	..	3.8	5.3	..	3.8	10.5	..	7.7	78.9	100.0	84.6	..	..	..
Hebephrenic	100.0	100.0	100.0	1.6	..	1.0	7.8	9.5	8.3	24.4	13.7	20.8	65.3	76.8	69.1	1.0	..	0.7
Catatonic	100.0	100.0	100.0	2.1	1.8	1.9	11.6	10.5	11.0	23.7	27.2	25.6	62.6	59.2	60.8	..	1.3	0.7
Paranoid	100.0	100.0	100.0	2.1	0.6	1.5	11.7	8.2	10.3	26.8	25.9	26.4	59.0	65.2	61.5	0.4	..	0.3
Others and unclassified	100.0	100.0	100.0	..	..	..	25.0	..	9.1	25.0	57.1	45.5	50.0	42.9	45.5	..	..	..
Total	100.0	100.0	100.0	2.0	1.0	1.6	10.4	9.3	9.9	24.7	24.2	24.5	62.5	64.8	63.5	0.5	0.6	0.5

TABLE 4. COMPARATIVE RATES OF RESULTS OF METRAZOL AND INSULIN TREATMENT ACCORDING TO TYPE OF DEMENTIA PRÆCOX

Type	Recovered		Much improved		Improved		Unimproved		Died	
	Metrazol	Insulin	Metrazol	Insulin	Metrazol	Insulin	Metrazol	Insulin	Metrazol	Insulin
Simple	3.8	4.2	3.8	41.7	7.7	37.5	84.6	16.7	...	...
Hebephrenic	1.0	6.3	8.3	25.7	20.8	20.9	69.1	46.1	0.7	1.0
Catatonic	1.9	17.4	11.0	25.6	25.6	27.0	60.8	29.5	0.7	0.6
Paranoid	1.5	12.7	10.3	28.1	26.4	25.7	61.5	31.5	0.3	2.0
Others and unclassified	..	20.0	9.1	40.0	45.5	...	45.5	40.0	...	...
Total	1.6	12.9	9.9	27.1	24.5	25.3	63.5	33.4	0.5	1.3

Age of Patients at Beginning of Treatment

Table 5 shows the outcome of metrazol treatment according to age at beginning of treatment. As would be expected the best results were obtained in the younger patients. None of the treated patients above 40 years of age were reported as recovered and only 6.1 per cent of the cases above 44 years of age were reported as much improved, compared with a general average rate of 9.9. Beyond the age of 25 there seems to be no close relationship between the improvement of the patients and their ages at beginning of treatment.

Duration of Psychosis Before Treatment

Table 6 shows the outcome of metrazol treatment according to duration of psychosis before treatment. Thirteen of the 18 recovered cases were treated within six months from the onset of the psychosis and 42 of the 113 much improved cases had a like duration of psychosis before treatment. It is noteworthy, however, that 203 of the 279 cases reported as improved had suffered with a psychosis from one to ten years. The table indicates that the probability of favorable results is much greater in the cases treated soon after the onset of the psychosis.

Duration of Treatment

The distribution of the treated patients by duration of treatment is shown in Table 7, together with the outcome for each period of treatment. It will be noted that of the 1,140 patients, 244 received treatment from 20 to 29 days, 197 from 40 to 49 days, 183 from 50 to 59 days, 176 from 60 to 69 days, and 107 from 70 to 79 days. There seems to be no close relationship between the period of treatment and the favorable results secured.

Injuries Sustained During Metrazol Treatment

A summary of injuries suffered by patients during metrazol treatment is shown by Table 8. Of the 1,140 patients treated, 87 were reported as suffering some injury during the course of treatment. Naturally the larger numbers of injured patients are reported by the hospitals treating the greater number of patients, although Creedmoor State Hospital reported but 5 injuries among

TABLE 5. OUTCOME OF METRAZOL TREATMENT ACCORDING TO AGE AT BEGINNING OF TREATMENT

Age group (years)	Total			Recovered			Much improved			Improved			Unimproved			Died		
	M.	F.	T.	M.	F.	T.	M.	F.	T.	M.	F.	T.	M.	F.	T.	M.	F.	T.
								Number										
10-14	1	1	2	..	..	..	..	..	..	1	1	2	..	..	..	..	..	..
15-19	30	35	65	1	2	3	6	4	10	11	8	19	12	21	33	..	..	..
20-24	150	79	229	5	1	6	23	9	32	31	13	44	91	56	147	..	..	..
25-29	193	112	305	2	2	4	13	10	23	46	23	69	132	76	208	..	1	1
30-34	153	133	286	3	..	3	12	10	22	40	35	75	96	87	183	2	1	3
35-39	80	67	147	2	..	2	6	6	12	24	20	44	48	40	88	..	1	1
40-44	31	42	73	..	..	..	5	7	12	5	14	19	20	21	41	1	..	1
45-49	6	21	27	..	..	..	2	..	2	1	5	6	3	16	19	..	..	..
50 and over	1	5	6	..	..	..	..	..	..	..	1	1	1	4	5	..	..	..
Total	645	495	1140	13	5	18	67	46	113	159	120	279	403	321	724	3	3	6
								Per Cent										
10-14	100.0	100.0	100.0	..	..	..	..	..	..	100.0	100.0	100.0	..	..	..	..	..	..
15-19	100.0	100.0	100.0	3.3	5.7	4.6	20.0	11.4	15.4	36.7	22.9	29.2	40.0	60.0	50.8	..	..	..
20-24	100.0	100.0	100.0	3.3	1.3	2.6	15.3	11.4	14.0	20.7	16.5	19.2	60.7	70.9	64.2	..	..	..
25-29	100.0	100.0	100.0	1.0	1.8	1.3	6.7	8.9	7.5	23.8	20.5	22.6	68.4	67.9	68.2	..	0.9	0.3
30-34	100.0	100.0	100.0	2.0	..	1.0	7.8	7.5	7.7	26.1	26.3	26.2	62.7	65.4	64.0	1.3	0.8	1.0
35-39	100.0	100.0	100.0	2.5	..	1.4	7.5	9.0	8.2	30.0	29.9	29.9	60.0	59.7	59.9	..	1.5	0.7
40-44	100.0	100.0	100.0	..	..	..	16.1	16.7	16.4	16.1	33.3	26.0	64.5	50.0	56.2	3.2	..	1.4
45-49	100.0	100.0	100.0	..	..	..	33.3	..	7.4	16.7	23.8	22.2	50.0	76.2	70.4	..	..	..
50 and over	100.0	100.0	100.0	..	..	..	..	..	..	..	20.0	16.7	100.0	80.0	83.3	..	..	..
Total	100.0	100.0	100.0	2.0	1.0	1.6	10.4	9.3	9.9	24.7	24.2	24.5	62.5	64.8	63.5	0.5	0.6	0.5

TABLE 6. OUTCOME OF METRAZOL TREATMENT ACCORDING TO DURATION OF PSYCHOSIS BEFORE TREATMENT

Total duration of psychosis	Total			Recovered			Much improved			Improved			Unimproved			Died		
	M.	F.	T.	M.	F.	T.	M.	F.	T.	M.	F.	T.	M.	F.	T.	M.	F.	T.
							Number											
Less than 1 month ...	3	13	16	..	1	1	1	4	5	2	3	5	..	5	5	..	..	..
1 to 3 months	31	31	62	5	3	8	14	10	24	8	8	16	4	10	14	..	..	..
4 to 6 months	31	26	57	4	..	4	7	6	13	9	12	21	11	8	19	..	..	..
7 to 12 months	29	34	63	1	..	1	11	7	18	8	14	22	9	12	21	..	1	1
1 to 2 years	156	143	299	2	1	3	20	11	31	54	38	92	79	92	171	1	1	2
3 to 5 years	199	136	335	1	..	1	7	5	12	50	21	71	141	109	250	..	1	1
6 to 10 years	142	90	232	..	..	..	7	3	10	22	18	40	112	69	181	1	..	1
11 to 14 years	34	13	47	..	..	..	..	..	..	4	5	9	30	8	38	..	..	..
15 to 19 years	10	5	15	..	..	..	..	..	..	..	1	1	9	4	13	1	..	1
20 years and over ...	10	4	14	..	..	..	..	..	..	2	..	2	8	4	12	..	..	..
Total	645	495	1140	13	5	18	67	46	113	159	120	279	403	321	724	3	3	6
							Per Cent											
Less than 1 month ...	100.0	100.0	100.0	..	7.7	6.3	33.3	30.8	31.3	66.7	23.1	31.3	..	38.5	31.3	..	..	..
1 to 3 months	100.0	100.0	100.0	16.1	9.7	12.9	45.2	32.3	38.7	25.8	25.8	25.8	12.9	32.3	22.6	..	..	..
4 to 6 months	100.0	100.0	100.0	12.9	..	7.0	22.6	23.1	22.8	29.0	46.2	36.8	35.5	30.8	33.3	..	..	..
7 to 12 months	100.0	100.0	100.0	3.4	..	1.6	37.9	20.6	28.6	27.6	41.2	34.9	31.0	35.3	33.3	..	2.9	1.6
1 to 2 years	100.0	100.0	100.0	1.3	0.7	1.0	12.8	7.7	10.4	34.6	26.6	30.8	50.6	64.3	57.2	0.6	0.7	0.7
3 to 5 years	100.0	100.0	100.0	0.5	..	0.3	3.5	3.7	3.6	25.1	15.4	21.2	70.9	80.1	74.6	..	0.7	0.3
6 to 10 years	100.0	100.0	100.0	..	..	..	4.9	3.3	4.3	15.5	20.0	17.2	78.9	76.7	78.0	0.7	..	0.4
11 to 14 years	100.0	100.0	100.0	..	..	..	..	..	..	11.8	38.5	19.1	88.2	61.5	80.9	..	..	..
15 to 19 years	100.0	100.0	100.0	..	..	..	..	..	..	..	20.0	6.7	90.0	80.0	86.7	10.0	..	6.7
20 years and over ...	100.0	100.0	100.0	..	..	..	..	..	..	20.0	..	14.3	80.0	100.0	85.7	..	..	..
Total	100.0	100.0	100.0	2.0	1.0	1.6	10.4	9.3	9.9	24.7	24.2	24.5	62.5	64.8	63.5	0.5	0.6	0.5

TABLE 7. OUTCOME OF METRAZOL TREATMENT ACCORDING TO DURATION OF TREATMENT

Duration of treatment, (days)	Total			Recovered			Much improved			Improved			Unimproved			Died		
	M.	F.	T.	M.	F.	T.	M.	F.	T.	M.	F.	T.	M.	F.	T.	M.	F.	T.
								Number										
Less than 10	14	8	22	..	..	..	..	1	1	1	1	2	13	5	18	..	1	1
10 to 19	24	32	56	1	3	4	6	2	8	3	6	9	14	21	35	..	..	..
20 to 29	155	89	244	3	..	3	4	8	12	20	12	32	128	68	196	..	1	1
30 to 39	39	35	74	3	..	3	8	9	17	9	6	15	19	20	39	..	..	..
40 to 49	62	135	197	3	1	4	10	7	17	12	45	57	36	82	118	1	..	1
50 to 59	105	78	183	1	1	2	7	6	13	22	16	38	74	54	128	1	1	2
60 to 69	115	61	176	1	..	1	7	7	14	40	18	58	67	36	103	..	..	..
70 to 79	73	34	107	..	..	..	17	3	20	25	10	35	31	21	52	..	..	..
80 to 89	34	9	43	1	..	1	6	2	8	13	2	15	13	5	18	1	..	1
90 to 99	9	5	14	..	..	..	1	..	1	7	..	7	1	5	6	..	..	..
100 and over	15	9	24	..	..	..	1	1	2	7	4	11	7	4	11	..	..	..
Total	645	495	1140	13	5	18	67	46	113	159	120	279	403	321	724	3	3	6
								Per Cent										
Less than 10	100.0	100.0	100.0	..	..	..	..	12.5	4.5	7.1	12.5	9.1	92.9	62.5	81.8	..	12.5	4.5
10 to 19	100.0	100.0	100.0	4.2	9.4	7.1	25.0	6.3	14.3	12.5	18.8	16.1	58.3	65.6	62.5	..	..	..
20 to 29	100.0	100.0	100.0	1.9	..	1.2	2.6	9.0	4.9	12.9	13.5	13.1	82.6	76.4	80.3	..	1.1	0.4
30 to 39	100.0	100.0	100.0	7.7	..	4.1	20.5	25.7	23.0	23.1	17.1	20.3	48.7	57.1	52.7	..	..	..
40 to 49	100.0	100.0	100.0	4.8	0.7	2.0	16.1	5.2	8.6	19.4	33.3	28.9	58.1	60.7	59.9	1.6	..	0.5
50 to 59	100.0	100.0	100.0	1.0	1.3	1.1	6.7	7.7	7.1	21.0	20.5	20.8	70.5	69.2	69.9	1.0	1.3	1.1
60 to 69	100.0	100.0	100.0	0.9	..	0.6	6.1	11.5	8.0	34.8	29.5	33.0	58.3	59.0	58.5	..	..	..
70 to 79	100.0	100.0	100.0	..	..	..	23.3	8.8	18.7	34.2	29.4	32.7	42.5	61.8	48.6	..	..	..
80 to 89	100.0	100.0	100.0	2.9	..	2.3	17.6	22.2	18.6	38.2	22.2	34.9	38.2	55.6	41.9	2.9	..	2.3
90 to 99	100.0	100.0	100.0	..	..	..	11.1	..	7.1	77.8	..	50.0	11.1	100.0	42.9	..	..	..
100 and over	100.0	100.0	100.0	..	..	..	6.7	11.1	8.3	46.7	44.4	45.8	46.7	44.4	45.8	..	..	..
Total	100.0	100.0	100.0	2.0	1.0	1.6	10.4	9.3	9.9	24.7	24.2	24.5	62.5	64.8	63.5	0.5	0.6	0.5

TABLE 8. INJURIES TO DEMENTIA PRÆCOX PATIENTS DURING METRAZOL TREATMENT

State hospitals	Total treated patients			Total injured patients			Dislocation of jaw			Fracture of jaw			Fractures of arms or shoulder			Fractures of legs			Dislocation of shoulder or arm			Other injuries		
	M.	F.	T.	M.	F.	T.	M.	F.	T.	M.	F.	T.	M.	F.	T.	M.	F.	T.	M.	F.	T.	M.	F.	T.
Brooklyn	135	194	329	8	14	22	8	12	20	..	..	..	..	..	..	..	..	..	..	1	1	..	1	1
Buffalo	24	22	46	3	2	5	..	1*	1	..	..	..	..	..	..	..	..	..	2	..	2	1	1	2
Central Islip	39	21	60	2	2	4	..	1	1	..	..	..	..	1	1	1	..	1	..	..	..	1	..	1
Creedmoor	81	40	121	3	2	5	..	2	2	..	..	..	..	..	..	..	..	..	..	..	..	3	..	3
Gowanda	43	28	71	4	2	6	1	1	2	..	..	..	..	1	1	..	..	..	2	..	2	1	..	1
Harlem Valley	..	2	2	..	..	..	..	..	..	..	..	..	..	..	..	..	..	..	..	..	..	..	..	..
Hudson River	33	32	65	4	7	11	4	6	10	..	..	..	..	..	..	..	..	..	..	..	..	..	1	1
Kings Park	35	20	55	3	1	4	..	..	..	1	..	1	..	..	..	..	..	..	..	..	..	2	1	3
Manhattan	13	15	28	..	..	..	..	..	..	..	..	..	..	..	..	..	..	..	..	..	..	..	..	..
Marcy	24	28	52	2	2	4	..	2	2	..	..	..	..	..	..	..	..	..	1	..	1	1	..	1
Pilgrim	2	1	3	2	..	2	2	..	2	..	..	..	..	..	..	..	..	..	..	..	..	..	..	..
Psychiatric Institute	11	3	14	..	..	..	1	..	1	..	..	..	..	..	..	..	..	..	..	..	..	..	1	1
Rockland	194	81	275	14	8	22	9	6	15	..	..	..	..	..	..	3	1	4	2	1	3	..	..	..
St. Lawrence	5	4	9	..	..	..	..	..	..	..	..	..	..	..	..	..	..	..	..	..	..	..	..	..
Utica	3	..	3	..	..	..	..	..	..	..	..	..	..	..	..	..	..	..	..	..	..	..	..	..
Willard	3	4	7	2	..	2	1	..	1	..	..	..	..	..	..	..	..	..	1	..	1	..	..	..
Total	645	495	1140	47	40	87	26	31	57	1	..	1	..	2	2	4	1	5	8	2	10	9	5	14

*Also dislocated shoulder.

121 patients treated. Brooklyn State Hospital reported 22 injured patients out of 329 treated. The corresponding numbers for Rockland State Hospital were 22 and 275. Hudson River State Hospital reported 11 injured patients out of 65 treated.

Of the 87 injured patients, 57 suffered dislocation of the jaw. Some of the patients suffered such dislocation several times, but no injured patient is counted more than once in the table. Fracture of the jaw occurred in 1 case, fracture of arms and shoulder in 2 cases and fracture of legs in 5 cases. Dislocation of shoulder or arms occurred in 10 cases and other injuries occurred in 14 cases.

It will be noted that of the 645 males 47 suffered injuries while of the 495 women 40 were injured. Six of the 1,140 patients, 3 men and 3 women, died during or following treatment.

Comment

The results of metrazol treatment shown in the foregoing statistical analysis raise grave doubts as to the wisdom of continuing this treatment in its current form as a routine procedure in the State hospitals. The data submitted show clearly the superiority of insulin treatment.

In certain cases in which insulin fails to yield favorable results metrazol perhaps may be found useful as a supplemental treatment.

The matter of injury to patients and the severity of the convulsions experienced by some of the patients treated are also worthy of consideration.

CHAPTER XIII

Mental Disease in Peru*

The care and treatment of the mentally ill in Peru have passed through a series of progressive stages similar to those undergone in the development of psychiatric service in the United States, Canada and various European countries. A long period of neglect was succeeded by inadequate almshouse or asylum care, which in turn was replaced by so-called hospital care with some degree of medical attention. With the general advance in psychiatry came the latest stage which embraces scientific treatment in a modern hospital with a competent staff of psychiatrists, nurses and attendants.

The first hospital provision for the care of mental patients in Peru was made in two general hospitals of Lima: the one, St. Andrew's Hospital for men; the other, St. Anna's Hospital for women. In each of these hospitals a special section was set apart for the care of mental patients. These sections were called "loquerias." The first mention of these was made by Father Juan Meléndez in 1678. He wrote concerning the "loqueria" in St. Andrew's Hospital which was used for the violent insane. He mentions one of the unfortunate disturbed patients who was put in a cage with his hands tied and was cared for by a charitable woman who cleaned the cage and gave him food and drink. Later in St. Peter's Hospital the violent insane were separated from the quiet cases. The former were chained while the latter were simply locked in cells. In the early part of the 19th century insane persons were less cruelly treated. They were kept in clean cells, bathed and given a certain degree of individual attention.

Toward the middle of the century the "loqueria" of St. Andrew's Hospital became in part an independent unit. It had its own budget and was called "Hospital Para Insanos." A special physician was provided to care for the mental patients. In 1857, the public welfare society† of Lima, which had charge of the hospital, appointed for this service Dr. José Casimiro Ulloa. Ulloa was an idealist. Upon investigation he found the "loquerias" of

*Published in American Journal of Psychiatry for September, 1939.

†Sociedad de Beneficencia Publica de Lima.

St. Andrew's and St. Anna's in bad condition and utterly inadequate for their purpose. He formed plans for needed improvements and sought aid in support of his projects. Fortunately, he was able to secure the active cooperation of the director of welfare, Don Francisco Carassa. With determination and persistence, the latter undertook the raising of funds for the erection of a suitable hospital for the patients who were unsatisfactorily cared for in the "loquerias." Success attended his efforts and eventually a large building was erected in the outskirts of Lima and was named "Hospital de la Misericordia." The new institution was opened December 16, 1859. It was considered a good asylum at the time. It had accommodations for 160 patients and soon after opening was caring for 153.

Naturally the new hospital used the means of treatment which prevailed at the time. These included surprise baths, baths for the disturbed similar to those used in the Salpêtrière, restraint chairs made in Paris, and wooden cribs or cages. There were also a variety of restraint apparatus, including iron bands for the feet and arms, to which chains were attached and fastened to the wall, strait jackets and barred cells. Many of these devices, silent witnesses of the ignorant cruelty of a bygone period, are still to be seen in the museum room of the Hospital Victor Larco Herrera in Lima.

The Hospital de la Misericordia was divided into four sections, the first for quiet cases; the second for those periodically disturbed; the third for mental defectives, epileptics and untidy cases; and the fourth for violent insane. This last section contained three strong cells such as were used in prisons.

Through the influence of Carassa and Ulloa the treatment of patients gradually improved. The policy of repression and restraint was modified and various activities were introduced to interest the patients and to provide an outlet for their energies.

Dr. Ulloa died in 1891 and was succeeded by Dr. Manuel A. Muniz, a physician who had studied in France and had observed the care of mental patients in other European countries. Muniz insisted on the use of gentle measures in caring for the insane and abolished all kinds of punishment. Although the original hospital had been enlarged, it had become crowded and antiquated. Dr. Muniz made plans for the erection of a new institution but died before his plans could be realized. He was succeeded by Dr. Matto, who was sent to Europe to study the organization of asylums for the insane. A site for the new institution was selected at Magdalena del Mar, about four miles from Lima. The building of the new hospital, however, was delayed, and it was not opened until 1918. Dr. Matto having died, Dr. Hermilio Valdizan was appointed resident physician and afterwards director of the hospital. Dr. Valdizan, who was a man of exceptional ability, became a leader in the advancement of psychiatric teaching and practice in his country.

The new hospital was made possible by a generous gift from Victor Larco Herrera, a philanthropist of Lima. Under the direction of Dr. Valdizan the institution made rapid progress and became a treatment hospital instead of a custodial asylum. Following the death of Dr. Valdizan in December, 1929, Dr. Baltazar Caravedo was appointed director of the hospital. He has continued the progressive policies of his predecessor.

On March 27, 1939, following the Pan American Neuropsychiatric Conference at Lima, Dr. Caravedo entertained the conference delegates at the hospital and showed them its facilities and activities. As it is the only hospital of its kind in Peru, it represents the standards of psychiatric service now in use in that country.

The Hospital Victor Larco Herrera

Bearing the name of its benefactor, Victor Larco Herrera, the Peruvian hospital for mental disease is located at Magdalena del Mar, a suburb of Lima, beautifully situated about four miles from the heart of the city. The year following its opening in 1918, the hospital cared for 817 patients. Since that time the number has increased from year to year until on the day of our visit, it had reached 1,315.

The hospital is built on the cottage plan. There are nine cottages for continued treatment cases and a reception cottage. Both private and public patients are cared for. Male private patients occupy one cottage and female private patients occupy two. The dependent patients occupy six cottages, three being devoted to the care of each sex. The reception building accommodates both males and females. In addition to the buildings mentioned, there is a small cottage for patients with infectious diseases; a cottage for the care of children of both sexes, most of whom are feebleminded; a cottage for physiotherapy; a mortuary; and an administration building. Separate homes are provided for the superintendent and steward. There is a nurses' home which also contains a sewing-room for the making of patients' clothing. No accommodations are provided for employees not engaged in ward work. A new cottage, which is nearly ready for occupancy, will care for the criminal insane.

In addition to the buildings mentioned, there are a well-equipped kitchen, a laundry, a bakery and various small buildings used for shops. Most of the cottages are one-story buildings. Some of those recently built, however, have two stories. The cottages as a whole constitute an attractive group but it is evident that strict economy was exercised in their construction. The kitchen is especially well adapted for its purpose. It is equipped with electric ranges and cookers which are said to give excellent service.

As the weather is warm throughout the year, no provision is made for heating any of the buildings.

The institution is well supplied with physicians, nurses and other employees. Including the superintendent, there are 12 physicians on the staff. Four of these are resident physicians. The others serve on part-time or are subject to call as their services are needed. One physician has charge of the laboratory and another of the physiotherapy cottage. A pharmacist and a part-time dentist are employed. The nursing force consists of the superintendent of nurses, two assistants to the superintendent, 58 ward nurses and 51 student nurses. Of the students, 32 are in the first year class, 11 in the second year class and 8 in the third year class. In addition to the employees mentioned there are 148 others who are engaged in conducting the general work of the institution. Counting pupil nurses as employees, the ratio of all employees to patients is 1 to 4; excluding pupil nurses, the ratio becomes 1 to 4.8.

The salaries and wages paid employees are very small compared to those prevalent in the United States. The money unit is the sol, which is worth about 20 cents in United States money. The superintendent receives an annual salary of 7,200 soles. The physicians receive salaries ranging from 1,200 to 3,000 soles. The salary of the superintendent of nurses is 3,600 soles and that of each assistant to the superintendent, 2,400. The salaries of other nurses run from 1,080 to 1,800 soles each. Physicians who lecture in the school of nursing are paid from 240 to 600 soles annually. Pupil nurses receive 20 soles per months during the first year, 30 the second year and 40 the third year.

The annual per capita cost of maintenance, exclusive of housing, of patients in this hospital is very low being approximately $110 in the year 1937.

The movement of patients in the hospital is extremely active. The hospital population on the 31st of December, 1936, was 1,123. The admissions during the year 1937 comprised 551 first admissions, 195 readmissions and 251 returns from parole, a total of 997. The departures during the year included 458 discharged patients, 264 paroled patients and 190 deaths, a total of 912, leaving a balance of 1,208 patients in the institution. In addition there were 157 on parole at the end of the year.

The ratio of first admissions and of patients under treatment to the general population of the country cannot be accurately computed as no general census of population has been taken in recent years. It is estimated, however, that the population of Peru is nearly 6,000,000. If this is correct, the ratio of mental patients to general population in this country is much lower than in the United States. Dr. Caravedo, the medical director, estimates the rate of resident patients per 100,000 of population to be 17. In New York State the rate is about 500. We are told, however, that the Peruvian hospital receives all patients sent to it and does not maintain a waiting list. Why such a small proportion of the people of Peru require treatment in mental hospitals is not answerable from available data.

In 1937, the Hospital Victor Larco Herrera introduced the revised classification of mental diseases which had been adopted by The American Psychiatric Association in 1934. The uniform statistical system of the association was brought into use at the same time. Through such action a comparison of mental diseases among first admissions in Peru and in the United States is now made possible. Of the 551 first admissions for the year 1937, 41, or 8.7 per cent, were classed in the syphilitic group; 53, or 11.2 per cent, in the alcoholic group; 32, or 6.8 per cent, in the epileptic group; 24, or 5.1 per cent, in the senile group; 33, or 7 per cent, in the manic-depressive group; 185, or 39.1 per cent in the dementia præcox group. Thirty-two psychotic patients were reported as undiagnosed.

Of the total first admissions, 78, or 14.2 per cent, were reported as without psychoses. Of these, 36 were classed as mental defectives. Comparing the above percentages with those found for first admissions in New York State, we note much higher percentages in Peru in dementia præcox and alcoholic cases, and much lower percentages in arteriosclerotic and senile cases. Apparently, arteriosclerotic cases are not freely sent to the mental hospital in Peru, as only 6 of the 551 first admissions were diagnosed as belonging to this group.

The Hospital Victor Larco Herrera, although serving as a public mental hospital for the whole country of Peru, is not maintained by national appropriation. The hospital is under the control of the "Sociedad de Beneficencia Publica de Lima." This welfare organization supplies funds necessary for maintenance of the institution and for additions and improvements. However, the hospital receives from the councils of the provinces and from the various departments of the national government funds for the maintenance of certain patients for whom these branches of government are responsible. In addition, the hospital receives pay for the maintenance of private patients. From these various sources were received 243,000 of the 633,000 soles expended for the maintenance of the institution in 1937.

A patient is admitted to the hospital on the application of his guardian, custodian or legal representative to the Sociedad de Beneficencia Publica de Lima. The application must state the reasons for the proposed commitment of the patient and must be accompanied by a certificate of one physician to the effect that the patient is mentally ill and in need of treatment in a mental hospital. If payment for the patient's maintenance is to be made, a contract therefor is entered into by his legal representative with the welfare society. Patients may also be committed by court order, police order or municipal council order by having prescribed forms filled out by authorized physicians and public officials. Provision is also made for the voluntary admission of suitable cases.

Treatment of patients in the Hospital Victor Larco Herrera has been modernized and at the present time compares favorably with that given in many mental hospitals of the United States.

When a patient is admitted to a hospital his personal and family history is compiled; he is given thorough psychiatric and physical examinations with such laboratory tests as may be indicated. Special treatment for physical disorders present is promptly instituted. After the patient has been under observation for a few weeks, his mental disorder is diagnosed and he is assigned to the ward most suitable for his treatment.

Seclusion and restraint are not used.

Patients are encouraged to work in the hospital industries and in the farm and garden but systematic occupational therapy has not been established.

Special treatment of schizophrenic patients by insulin and metrazol was introduced in 1937 and has been continued since that time. Favorable results from the use of both drugs are reported.

A commendable feature of treatment not ordinarily found in mental hospitals is the practice in use here of giving every patient a physical reexamination every three months and a psychiatric reexamination every six months. These examinations are of much value in adjusting treatment to the needs of the individual patient.

Social workers connected with the outpatient department are employed to find suitable places for patients who are ready for parole, and to exercise a certain degree of supervision over patients placed on parole. Patients who have recovered or have improved so that they may live safely in the community are either definitely or conditionally discharged. The conditional discharge is practically a trial leave of absence or parole, and must terminate at the end of three months by definite discharge or by return to the hospital. Court cases may be discharged only on the authorization of the committing magistrate. In 1937, the hospital discharged 76 as recovered and 261 as improved. The rates based on all admissions were 10.2 and 35.0 per cent, respectively.

Mental Hygiene Activities in Peru

Preventive mental hygiene work in Peru is of recent date and is not yet well developed. It consists of two principal activities; first, the publication and dissemination of information concerning mental hygiene, and second, clinic work for both adults and children. The general instruction of the population in mental hygiene is difficult because of the types of people that must be dealt with. More than half of the population of Peru consists of native Peruvians commonly called Indians. The remainder of the population is composed of white people, mostly of Spanish or Italian descent; mixed races representing an amalgamation of Europeans and natives; a considerable number of Negroes and some Chinese and Japanese. A large part of the Indian population does not utilize the services of trained physicians but still uses the primitive treatment methods that were developed during their tribal life. Sorcery and magic have a large place in such methods. Various herbs are used in connection with the magic rites of the medicine men. As nervous and mental diseases are not understood by these primitive people, they are treated by various forms of magic. Among part of the mixed population the ideas of the Indians with respect to the treatment of disease still prevail, but in the main the mixed peoples are more ready to engage the services of physicians when they become seriously ill. This part of the population, however, has very little knowledge of the nature of mental disease and is not inclined to seek the aid of physicians or psychiatrists when relatives become mentally afflicted. The white peoples, although they have had little opportunity to become familiar with psychiatric practice or mental hygiene, are more ready to accept and use new ideas and methods developed by medical science.

Through the efforts of Dr. Honorio Delgado and Dr. H. Valdizan, a propaganda campaign was inaugurated in 1919 for the teaching of mental hygiene to the medical profession. A series of conferences was held in which various aspects of mental health were discussed. These discussions were arranged by an organization known as "Seminario Psicopedagógico," and were attended largely by physicians and educational leaders. In 1922, the first conference on the Peruvian child was held. At this time Doctors Valdizan and Delgado proposed the creation in Peru of a national mental hygiene league. It was hoped that such an organization would function like the mental hygiene committees of the United States and other countries. The league was organized and prepared, in its first year, a pamphlet on mental hygiene which was published by the "Sociedad de Beneficencia Publica de Lima." The later official recognition of the league is due largely to Dr. M. Caravedo, who since 1932 has published a mental hygiene periodical known as "Boletin de Higiene Mental."

To further aid in the dissemination of mental hygiene principles, Dr. H. Delgado wrote and published in 1922 a small book entitled "Some Aspects of the Psychology of the Child." This book contained an introduction by the late Dr. William A. White of Washington, D. C. In 1933, Dr. Delgado published another book, entitled "The Mental Development of the Individual."

About 1920 mental hygiene clinics were begun by Dr. Delgado in the Hospital Victor Larco Herrera. These at first consisted of free consultations offered to outpatients by physicians of the hospital. During recent years the clinic work has expanded and at the present time the clinic visits each year number several hundred.

Considerable work has also been done for the prevention of juvenile delinquency. A children's court was organized in 1925 and an organization for the protection of children in 1928. In this work Mrs. M. G. Parks has had a large part. Some years ago she made a study of the work of the Bureau of Child Guidance of the National Committee for Mental Hygiene of New York and of the Judge Baker Foundation in Boston, and has adapted, so far as possible, the methods of these organizations in dealing with the children of Lima. The problem children referred to the protective society are carefully studied and are placed, so far as possible, in proper homes and are supervised for a period averaging more than one year.

The leading organizations of Lima are taking an active interest in child guidance and Dr. Delgado in 1920 formulated a child guidance program, at the request of the Minister of Justice and Education. The program was submitted to the Peruvian Congress but was not adopted.

The psychiatric leaders of Peru clearly recognize that the single mental hospital of Peru is not large enough to accommodate the mental cases of that country that should receive hospital treatment. The hospital is now crowded beyond capacity and funds are not at present available for its enlargement. In order to meet the situation adequately, it is felt that a new hospital should be established in southern Peru, probably at Arequipa, and later a third hospital should be built to accommodate the people of northern Peru. It seems certain that with the gradual enlightenment of the population, the demand for hospital treatment of mental diseases will be greatly increased. It is also probable that with the psychiatric progress that Lima is now making, means will be found for the establishment of necessary institutions for the treatment of mental disorders.

BIBLIOGRAPHY

Delgado, H.: La psychiatrie et l'hygiene mentale au Perou. L'Hygiene mentale, journal de psychiatrie appliquée, 8:121-200, Paris, 1936.

Caravedo, B.: Memoria de la direccion de Hospital Victor Larco Herrara. Peru, 1937.

——: Victor Larco Herrera Hospital. Nosokomeion, X, 1:64-67, Stuttgart, Germany, 1939.

CHAPTER XIV

Use and Effect of Alcohol in Relation to Alcoholic Mental Disease Before, During and After Prohibition*

Because of its prevalence and its preventability, alcoholic mental disease is of special social interest. Such interest has been taken into account by the statistical bureau of the New York State Department of Mental Hygiene in its annual compilation of data concerning mental diseases since 1913. In addition to the usual statistical information concerning all first admissions, a special schedule report for each alcoholic case has been required from the State hospitals. The supplementary questions on the schedule relating to the use and effect of alcohol are as follows:

1. At what age did patient become addicted to the use of alcoholic liquors?
2. What liquors did patient drink? To which was he especially addicted?
3. Was patient a regular or a periodic drinker? What quantity of liquor did he drink?
4. Did patient become intoxicated? If so, how often?
5. Did patient's drinking cause him to lose time from his regular occupation? If so, to what extent?
6. Did patient's drinking affect his general health? If so, how?
7. Has patient had delirium tremens? If so, how many times?
8. Has patient had previous attacks of alcoholic mental disease?
9. Did he use drugs? If so, specify kind, and extent of use.
10. Was alcohol the principal or contributory cause of patient's insanity?

The data reported in answer to these questions for the fiscal year ended September 30, 1914, were tabulated by the author and published in the *State Hospital Bulletin* for August, 1915, under the title *The Use and Effect of Alcohol in Relation to the Alcoholic Psychoses.* In the year 1914, a considerable number of the rural districts of the State had become dry under local option laws, and for the preceding two years there had been a slight decline in the rate of alcoholic first admissions. The group studied at that time comprised 464 first admissions.

As important changes in Federal and State regulation of the liquor traffic have taken place since 1914, it was deemed desirable to make a comparative study of later periods. The periods chosen for such study comprise (1) the years 1920-1923, inclusive,

*Published in Mental Hygiene for January, 1940.

TABLE 1. AGE AT WHICH DRINK HABIT WAS ACQUIRED, FIRST ADMISSIONS OF 1920-1923

Type of alcoholic psychosis	Total			Under 20 years			20-24 years			25-29 years			30-34 years			35-39 years			40-44 years			45-49 years			50 years and over			Unascertained		
	M.	F.	T.	M.	F.	T.	M.	F.	T.	M.	F.	T.	M.	F.	T.	M.	F.	T.	M.	F.	T.	M.	F.	T.	M.	F.	T.	M.	F.	T.
Pathological intoxication ...	44	13	57	18*	4	22	9	1	10	9	1	10	1	..	1	1	..	1	..	1	1	..	..	..	..	..	..	6	6	12
Delirium tremens	50	11	61	23**	3	26	13	2	15	2	..	2	2	1	3	1	3	4	..	..	..	..	..	..	..	..	..	9	2	11
Korsakow's psychosis	46	12	58	19†	..	19	9	4	13	3	1	4	2	..	2	..	2	2	1	..	1	..	1	1	3	..	3	9	4	13
Acute hallucinosis	252	38	290	109	4	113	58	5	63	14	5	19	16	3	19	2	6	8	3	1	4	..	..	..	..	..	..	50	14	64
Alcoholic deterioration	23	14	37	11	2	13	6	3	9	3	..	3	1	2	3	..	1	1	..	..	..	..	..	..	..	1	1	2	5	7
Paranoid states	82	11	93	29	3	32	26	2	28	6	2	8	3	1	4	2	1	3	1	..	1	..	..	..	1	..	1	14	2	16
Confusional states	11	5	16	5	1	6	3	1	4	2	..	2	..	1	1	..	1	1	..	..	..	..	..	..	..	..	..	1	1	2
Other types	36	14	50	8	1	9	13	2	15	2	5	7	2	2	4	..	..	..	..	..	..	..	..	..	2	..	2	9	4	13
Total	544	118	662	222	18	240	137	20	157	41	14	55	27	10	37	6	14	20	5	2	7	..	1	1	6	1	7	100	38	138

*One at three years of age in Russia.
**One at eight years.
†One at seven, another at ten.

TABLE 2. AGE AT WHICH DRINK HABIT WAS ACQUIRED, FIRST ADMISSIONS OF 1936-1937

Type of alcoholic psychosis	Total			Under 20 years			20-24 years			25-29 years			30-34 years			35-39 years			40-44 years			45-49 years			50 years and over			Unascertained		
	M.	F.	T.	M.	F.	T.	M.	F.	T.	M.	F.	T.	M.	F.	T.	M.	F.	T.	M.	F.	T.	M.	F.	T.	M.	F.	T.	M.	F.	T.
Pathological intoxication ..	120	23	143	23	5	28	15	4	19	10	2	12	7	1	8	4	3	7	3	2	5	1	1	2	1	2	3	56	3	59
Delirium tremens	211	41	252	58	4	62	44	4	48	20	4	24	9	6	15	5	6	11	3	4	7	4	..	4	..	2	2	68	11	79
Korsakow's psychosis	127	50	177	27	4	31	31	..	31	14	3	17	9	9	18	3	5	8	2	1	3	1	5	6	2	5	7	38	18	56
Acute hallucinosis	294	54	348	77	7	84	88	8	96	38	14	52	13	8	21	10	3	13	9	3	12	2	1	3	3	2	5	54	8	62
Alcoholic deterioration ...	188	63	251	49	5	54	50	9	59	24	7	31	9	11	20	5	7	12	3	2	5	4	4	8	1	2	3	43	16	59
Paranoid states	125	24	149	26	6	32	38	3	41	18	1	19	6	1	7	3	2	5	6	4	10	2	2	4	3	..	3	23	5	28
Confusional states	123	29	152	49	..	49	34	5	39	15	3	18	6	1	7	4	1	5	4	3	7	4	1	5	2	1	3	5	14	19
Other	81	33	114	21	4	25	22	1	23	7	9	16	10	3	13	4	6	10	1	1	2	1	1	2	4	3	7	11	5	16
Total	1,269	317	1,586	330	35	365	322	34	356	146	43	189	69	40	109	38	33	71	31	20	51	19	15	34	16	17	33	298	80	378

and (2) the years 1936-1937, inclusive. The first period covered four years of comparatively effective prohibition, and the second period, two years under State and local regulation. The difference in the numbers of first admissions in the two periods is striking, the four years under prohibition yielding only 817 alcoholic first admissions, or an average of 204 per year, as compared with 1,703, or an average of 852 per year in the two years under the present license system.

As satisfactory answers to the questions on the schedule were unobtainable in many cases, it became necessary to limit the tabulation to 662 first admissions in the first period and to 1,586 in the second. In tabulating the data, the several questions were taken up in order. The cases were separated by sex and type of alcoholic psychoses so that the relations of each sex and of the various types with respect to the use of alcohol could be more clearly seen.

Question 1.—*At what age did patient become addicted to the use of alcoholic liquors?*

The data reported in answer to this question are presented in Tables 1-4. It is clear from the answers that the drink habit resulting in alcoholic mental disease is formed early in life. Naturally, many of the answers lacked definiteness, as precise information was not available. In the following comparisons the percentages are based on ascertained cases.

In the 1914 study, 45.5 per cent of the males and 12.5 of the females were under twenty when the drink habit was formed. In the 1920-1923 period, the corresponding percentages were 50.0 and 22.5, and in the 1936-1937 period, 34.0 and 14.8. The female patients at the time of the formation of the drink habit were on the average older than the male in all three periods. The comparative figures for the ascertained cases were:

Average Age at Formation of Drink Habit

Period	Males	Females
1914	21.4	27.9
1920-23	20.6	25.8
1936-37	23.9	31.7

It will be observed that the 1920-1923 group were younger than the other groups when the drink habit was formed.

The average ages of the patients of the three groups at time of admission were not widely divergent; however, the 1936-1937 group averaged about two years older than the other groups. The following are the comparative figures:

Average Age on Admission

Period	Males	Females
1914	43.6	44.3
1920-23	43.9	43.3
1936-37	45.9	45.8

Among males the average duration of the drink habit prior to admission in the 1936-1937 group was 22 years and among females 14.1 years. These data have great significance from the point of view of preventive effort. During the long period of excessive drinking that precedes the onset of alcoholic mental disorder, it should be possible to check the habit and protect the alcoholic so that mental disease might be averted.

TABLE 3. AVERAGE AGE AT TIME OF ADMISSION OF ALCOHOLIC PATIENTS AND AVERAGE DURATION OF DRINK HABIT BEFORE ADMISSION, FIRST ADMISSIONS OF 1920-1923

Type of alcoholic psychosis	Average age at admission			Average duration of drink habit, in years		
	Males	Females	Total	Males	Females	Total
Pathological intoxication ...	40.8	43.1	41.3	20.2	19.7	20.2
Delirium tremens	41.9	39.8	41.6	22.0	12.9	20.4
Korsakow's psychosis	53.4	43.8	51.4	31.2	16.4	28.5
Acute hallucinosis	41.4	42.3	41.5	21.6	15.6	21.0
Alcoholic deterioration	47.4	45.2	46.3	27.1	16.3	24.0
Paranoid states	45.9	42.8	45.6	25.0	20.4	24.5
Confusional states	48.6	51.8	49.6	26.3	29.7	27.3
Other types	46.5	44.9	46.0	22.6	18.8	21.5
Total	43.9	43.3	43.7	23.3	17.5	22.4

It will be noted in Tables 3 and 4 that marked differences among patients of the several types are shown in the average age on admission and in the average duration of the drink habit. The Korsakow group was the oldest in both periods and had the longest average duration of the drink habit in the 1920-1923 period. The acute-hallucinosis group was the youngest in the 1936-1937 period. Patients of each type averaged about forty years of age in both periods. All types gave a history of from fourteen to twenty-eight years of excessive drinking prior to admission.

TABLE 4. AVERAGE AGE AT TIME OF ADMISSION OF ALCOHOLIC PATIENTS AND AVERAGE DURATION OF DRINK HABIT BEFORE ADMISSION, FIRST ADMISSIONS OF 1936-1937

Type of alcoholic psychosis	Average age at admission			Average duration of drink habit, in years		
	Males	Females	Total	Males	Females	Total
Pathological intoxication ...	44.6	45.2	44.7	17.8	15.8	17.3
Delirium tremens	43.2	42.2	43.0	20.0	13.5	18.9
Korsakow's psychosis	51.2	49.1	50.6	28.0	12.0	23.7
Acute hallucinosis	41.9	37.7	41.2	18.2	8.7	16.6
Alcoholic deterioration	48.8	49.6	49.0	24.4	18.8	23.0
Paranoid states	48.0	45.4	47.6	23.0	15.1	21.8
Confusional states	49.5	52.3	50.1	26.3	20.7	25.7
Other types	46.0	49.8	46.2	21.2	12.5	18.8
Total	45.9	45.8	45.9	22.0	14.1	20.4

Question 2.—What liquors did patient drink? To which was he especially addicted?

The tabulated answers are given in Tables 5 and 6.

Whiskey stands out as by far the most common alcoholic drink indulged in by these patients. Of the 1920-1923 group, 66.4 per cent drank whiskey to excess, and of the 1936-1937 group, the percentage was 76.6. The percentage of cases drinking beer only was 16.9 in the former group and 7.4 in the latter. These two beverages were both indulged in by many patients and several other combinations of drinks were reported. The choice of beverages by males and females was in general quite similar.

In 1914, 47.2 per cent of the alcoholic cases were addicted to whiskey and 33.6 per cent to beer. Apparently in the later years whiskey had become a more potent cause of alcoholic mental disease.

TABLE 5. KINDS OF LIQUOR TO WHICH PATIENTS WERE ESPECIALLY ADDICTED, FIRST ADMISSIONS OF 1920-1923

Type of alcoholic psychosis	Total			Whiskey and alcohol		Whiskey and beer		Wine only		Beer only*		All others		Unascertained	
	M.	F.	T.	M.	F.	M.	F.	M.	F.	M.	F.	M.	F.	M.	F.
Pathological intoxication	44	13	57	26	8	3	..	3	1	10	1	2	2	..	1
Delirium tremens	50	11	61	37	5	3	1	..	4	6	1	2	..	2	..
Korsakow's psychosis	46	12	58	32	6	3	..	..	..	6	2	2	1	3	3
Acute hallucinosis	252	38	290	152	21	15	..	17	1	42	5	15	7	11	4
Alcoholic deterioration	23	14	37	17	9	2	..	..	..	3	1	..	2	1	2
Paranoid states	82	11	93	52	7	4	1	2	1	15	1	4	1	5	..
Confusional states	11	5	16	6	5	..	..	..	..	3	..	2	..	..	..
Other	36	14	50	26	8	..	..	..	..	7	3	1	3	2	..
Total	544	118	662	348	69	30	2	22	7	92	14	28	16	24	10

*Includes ales.

TABLE 6. KINDS OF LIQUOR TO WHICH PATIENTS WERE ESPECIALLY ADDICTED, FIRST ADMISSIONS OF 1936-1937

Type of alcoholic psychosis	Total			Whiskey and alcohol		Whiskey and beer		Wine only		Beer only		All others		Unascertained	
	M.	F.	T.	M.	F.	M.	F.	M.	F.	M.	F.	M.	F.	M.	F.
Pathological intoxication	120	23	143	86	14	16	1	..	2	7	3	6	2	5	1
Delirium tremens	211	41	252	162	32	18	..	1	1	12	3	8	..	10	5
Korsakow's psychosis	127	50	177	90	28	11	3	1	3	8	5	4	7	13	4
Acute hallucinosis	294	54	348	214	41	25	1	6	1	21	5	15	3	13	3
Alcoholic deterioration	188	63	251	154	43	15	5	1	2	5	9	6	3	7	1
Paranoid states	125	24	149	87	14	12	4	9	2	9	1	8	3	..	..
Confusional states	123	29	152	95	23	7	2	3	1	10	1	6	1	2	1
Other	81	33	114	63	18	5	3	..	2	7	5	4	5	2	..
Total	1,269	317	1,586	951	213	109	19	21	14	79	32	57	24	52	15

Question 3.—Was the patient a regular or periodic drinker? What quantity of liquor did he drink?

Tables 7 and 8 give the tabulated answers.

TABLE 7. NATURE OF DRINK HABIT, FIRST ADMISSIONS OF 1920-1923

Type of alcoholic psychosis	Total			Regular			Periodic			Unascertained		
	M.	F.	T.	M.	F.	T.	M.	F.	T.	M.	F.	T.
Pathological intoxication	44	13	57	26	11	37	17	1	18	1	1	2
Delirium tremens	50	11	61	37	9	46	13	2	15	..	..	..
Korsakow's psychosis ..	46	12	58	32	10	42	14	2	16	..	..	..
Acute hallucinosis	252	38	290	165	26	191	83	12	95	4	..	4
Alcoholic deterioration..	23	14	37	20	10	30	2	3	5	1	1	2
Paranoid states	82	11	93	66	11	77	16	..	16	..	..	..
Confusional states	11	5	16	7	4	11	4	1	5	..	..	..
Other types	36	14	50	25	10	35	11	2	13	..	2	2
Total	544	118	662	378	91	469	160	23	183	6	4	10

TABLE 8. NATURE OF DRINK HABIT, FIRST ADMISSIONS OF 1936-1937

Type of alcoholic psychosis	Total			Regular			Periodic			Unascertained		
	M.	F.	T.	M.	F.	T.	M.	F.	T.	M.	F.	T.
Pathological intoxication	120	23	143	60	10	70	41	13	54	19	..	19
Delirium tremens	211	41	252	119	32	151	73	9	82	19	..	19
Korsakow's psychosis ..	127	50	177	99	40	139	18	7	25	10	3	13
Acute hallucinosis	294	54	348	162	39	201	120	14	134	12	1	13
Alcoholic deterioration..	188	63	251	135	44	179	51	18	69	2	1	3
Paranoid states	125	24	149	84	18	102	39	6	45	2	..	2
Confusional states	123	29	152	77	19	96	46	10	56	..	..	..
Other types	81	33	114	40	22	62	40	10	50	1	1	2
Total	1,269	317	1,586	776	224	1,000	428	87	515	65	6	71

Of the 652 ascertained cases of the 1920-1923 group, 469, or 71.9 per cent, drank regularly, and 183, or 28.1 per cent, drank periodically. Of the 1,515 patients of the 1936-1937 group whose drinking habits were reported, 1,000, or 66.0 per cent, were regular drinkers and 515, or 34 per cent, were periodic drinkers. In 1914, the regular drinkers constituted 77.8 per cent of the total.

Among both regular and periodic drinkers a fixed habit of excessive drinking was indicated. Many of the regular drinkers consumed large quantities of liquor every day, some as much as two or three quarts of whiskey. The periodic drinkers would abstain or drink moderately for a week or a month and then throw restraint aside and enter on a period of debauch.

No marked differences in the drinking habits of the patients of the several types are noted. As would be expected, in the 1920-1923 period, home-brewed beer and moonshine whiskey were frequently substituted for commercial products.

Excess in drinking is further indicated by the frequency of intoxication which was reported in answer to the next question.

Question 4.—*Did patient become intoxicated? If so, how often?*

Satisfactory information with reference to the fact of intoxication was obtained for 645 of the 662 cases of the 1920-1923 period, and for 1,139 of the 1,586 cases of 1936-1937 period. Only 34, or 5.3 per cent, of the first group, and 51, or 4.5 per cent, of the second group were reported as not having been intoxicated. Of the 1914 cases, the corresponding percentage was 12.7. The frequency of intoxication of the patients included in the present study was irregular in many cases. A large proportion of the patients of both periods became intoxicated once a week or oftener. A spree at the week end or after pay day was a common occurrence.

Question 5.—*Did patient's drinking cause him to lose time from his regular employment? If so, to what extent?*

The data on this point are presented in Tables 9 and 10.

Reliable information concerning loss of time from employment was not obtainable in 56 cases of the 1920-1923 group and in 354 cases of the 1936-1937 group. Among the ascertained cases of the former group, no loss of time was reported for 322, or 53.1 per cent. For the latter group, the corresponding number was 587, or 47.6 per cent. In 1914, the percentage of cases suffering no loss of time was 35.1. Many other cases of all three periods were not so fortunate. Loss of position was suffered by 29, or 4.8 per cent, of the patients of the 1920-1923 group, and by 209, or 17.0 per cent, of the 1936-1937 group. In 1914, such loss was suffered by 25.4 per cent of the ascertained cases. When the heavy drinking is taken into consideration, one would expect even larger losses.

TABLE 9. LOSS OF EMPLOYMENT, FIRST ADMISSIONS OF 1920-1923

Type of alcoholic psychosis	Total			No loss			Occasionally a day			Several days a month			Loss of position			Indefinite loss of work*			Unascertained		
	M.	F.	T.	M.	F.	T.	M.	F.	T.	M.	F.	T.	M.	F.	T.	M.	F.	T.	M.	F.	T.
Pathological intoxication	44	13	57	26	5	31	4	1	5	5	..	5	..	..	..	5	7	12	4	..	4
Delirium tremens	50	11	61	27	4	31	5	1	6	6	..	6	1	..	1	8	4	12	3	2	5
Korsakow's psychosis	46	12	58	19	7	26	2	..	2	6	..	6	4	..	4	11	2	13	4	3	7
Acute hallucinosis	252	38	290	125	17	142	29	..	29	35	3	38	13	1	14	30	11	41	20	6	26
Alcoholic deterioration	23	14	37	5	6	11	1	2	3	..	..	..	3	1	4	12	4	16	2	1	3
Paranoid states	82	11	93	38	7	45	4	..	4	6	..	6	5	..	5	23	3	26	6	1	7
Confusional states	11	5	16	7	1	8	2	..	2	1	2	3	..	..	..	1	2	3	..	..	..
Other types	36	14	50	21	7	28	5	1	6	2	..	2	1	..	1	4	5	9	3	1	4
Total	544	118	662	268	54	322	52	5	57	61	5	66	27	2	29	94	38	132	42	14	56

*Includes neglect of home.

TABLE 10. LOSS OF EMPLOYMENT, FIRST ADMISSIONS OF 1936-1937

Type of alcoholic psychosis	Total			No loss			Occasionally a day			Several days a month			Loss of position			Indefinite loss of work			Unascertained		
	M.	F.	T.	M.	F.	T.	M.	F.	T.	M.	F.	T.	M.	F.	T.	M.	F.	T.	M.	F.	T.
Pathological intoxication	120	23	143	31	6	37	5	..	5	3	1	4	11	4	15	17	6	23	53	6	59
Delirium tremens	211	41	252	83	14	97	2	3	5	9	..	9	29	..	29	34	13	47	54	11	65
Korsakow's psychosis	127	50	177	37	13	50	..	..	..	2	3	5	19	4	23	33	21	54	36	9	45
Acute hallucinosis	294	54	348	126	23	149	4	..	4	8	1	9	36	8	44	65	11	76	55	11	66
Alcoholic deterioration	188	63	251	49	22	71	..	..	..	5	2	7	39	4	43	46	26	72	49	9	58
Paranoid states	125	24	149	58	3	61	3	..	3	1	..	1	20	1	21	23	12	35	20	8	28
Confusional states	123	29	152	68	11	79	..	..	..	3	..	3	16	2	18	29	5	34	7	11	18
Other types	81	33	114	31	12	43	3	..	3	1	1	2	13	3	16	24	11	35	9	6	15
Total	1,269	317	1,586	483	104	587	17	3	20	32	8	40	183	26	209	271	105	376	283	71	354

Question 6.—*Did patient's drinking affect his general health? If so, how?*

The first part of this question was answered in the affirmative for 226, or 35.9 per cent, of the ascertained cases of the 1920-1923 group. The corresponding figures for the 1936-1937 group was 536, or 37.1 per cent. In 1914, the percentage was 40.1.

A large proportion of the patients of all three groups were afflicted with physical disorders, many of which were of long standing. The extent to which alcohol caused, or contributed to, these disorders cannot be definitely determined.

Question 7.—*Has patient had delirium tremens? If so, how many times?*

Tables 11 and 12 give the data reported.

Reliable information concerning the occurrence of delirium tremens was obtained in 597 cases of the 1920-1923 group and in 1,457 cases of the 1936-1937 group. A negative history of the disorder was obtained in 457, or 76.5 per cent, of the 1920-1923 group, and in 1,028, or 70.6 per cent. of the 1936-1937 group. A positive history was obtained in 140, or 23.5 per cent, of the former group, and in 429, or 29.4 per cent, of the latter group.

Of the 140 positive cases of the 1920-1923 group, 101 had had one attack, 23 had had two, 7 had had three, and 9 had had more than three attacks. Of the 429 positive cases of the 1936-1937 group, the numbers with one, two, and three or more attacks were 349, 29, 23, and 28, respectively.

Question 8.—*Has patient had previous attacks of alcoholic mental disease?*

Information concerning previous attacks of alcoholic mental disease was obtained in 648 cases of the 1920-1923 group and in 1,561 cases of the 1936-1937 group. The question was answered affirmatively in 81 cases of the former group and in 221 cases of the latter group.

Question 9.—*Did patient use drugs? If so, specify kind and extent of use.*

The habits of the patients with respect to the use of narcotic drugs were ascertained in 639 cases of the 1920-1923 group and in

TABLE 11. FREQUENCY OF DELIRIUM TREMENS, FIRST ADMISSIONS OF 1920-1923

Type of alcoholic psychosis	Total			At least once			Twice			Three times			More than three times			Not at all			Unascertained		
	M.	F.	T.	M.	F.	T.	M.	F.	T.	M.	F.	T.	M.	F.	T.	M.	F.	T.	M.	F.	T.
Pathological intoxication	44	13	57	5	1	6	2	..	2	..	..	..	2	..	2	31	10	41	4	2	6
Delirium tremens	50	11	61	42	11	53	5	..	5	1	..	1	2	..	2	..	..	..	..	..	..
Korsakow's psychoses	46	12	58	5	1	6	2	..	2	..	..	..	..	..	..	28	9	37	11	2	13
Acute hallucinosis	252	38	290	16	5	21	11	..	11	4	..	4	4	..	4	198	27	225	19	6	25
Alcoholic deterioration	23	14	37	3	..	3	1	..	1	..	..	..	..	..	..	15	10	25	4	4	8
Paranoid states	82	11	93	4	1	5	..	1	1	1	..	1	..	..	..	67	9	76	10	..	10
Confusional states	11	5	16	2	1	3	..	..	..	..	..	..	..	..	..	9	4	13	..	..	..
Other types	36	14	50	2	2	4	..	1	1	1	..	1	1	..	1	29	11	40	3	..	3
Total	544	118	662	79	22	101	21	2	23	7	..	7	9	..	9	377	80	457	51	14	65

TABLE 12. FREQUENCY OF DELIRIUM TREMENS, FIRST ADMISSIONS OF 1936-1937

Type of alcoholic psychosis	Total			At least once			Twice			Three times			More than three times			Not at all			Unascertained		
	M.	F.	T.	M.	F.	T.	M.	F.	T.	M.	F.	T.	M.	F.	T.	M.	F.	T.	M.	F.	T.
Pathological intoxication	120	23	143	9	1	10	..	..	..	1	..	1	4	..	4	88	20	108	18	2	20
Delirium tremens	211	41	252	190	38	228	10	..	10	6	2	8	5	1	6	..	..	..	..	..	..
Korsakow's psychosis	127	50	177	13	5	18	2	..	2	4	..	4	3	..	3	77	32	109	28	13	41
Acute hallucinosis	294	54	348	33	6	39	9	..	9	5	..	5	6	..	6	221	45	266	20	3	23
Alcoholic deterioration	188	63	251	22	10	32	3	1	4	2	1	3	1	1	2	147	43	190	13	7	20
Paranoid states	125	24	149	9	1	10	1	1	2	1	..	1	2	1	3	103	21	124	9	..	9
Confusional states	123	29	152	5	..	5	..	..	..	1	..	1	3	1	4	107	26	133	7	2	9
Other types	81	33	114	6	1	7	2	..	2	..	..	..	..	..	..	68	30	98	5	2	7
Total	1,269	317	1,586	287	62	349	27	2	29	20	3	23	24	4	28	811	217	1,028	100	29	129

1,549 cases of the 1936-1937 group. The drug users comprised 17 males and 11 females of the former group and 29 males and 27 females of the latter group. It is apparent from the data that drug addiction was not a common accompaniment of the alcoholic addiction and was not a large factor in the development of the alcoholic mental disorder.

Question 10.—*Was alcohol the principal or a contributory cause of the patient's mental disease?*

Alcohol was reported as the principal cause of the patient's mental disease in 633 of the 649 ascertained cases of the 1920-1923 group and in 1,535 of the 1,570 ascertained cases of the 1936-1937 group.

A further question as to the cause of the patient's inebriety was asked, but the information obtained was not considered adequate for tabulation.

Comment and Conclusions

From the data presented in this paper, the following conclusions seem warranted:

1. The onset of alcoholic mental disease, as a rule, occurs only after several years of excessive drinking. The period for male patients averages about twenty-two years and for female patients about fifteen years.

2. The average age of alcoholic patients on admission to a State mental hospital is approximately forty-five years. The fact that alcoholic mental disease occurs in the most productive period of life adds greatly to its economic and social significance.

3. Whiskey and beer are the principal beverages that cause alcoholic mental disease. Of the two, whiskey, either alone or in combination, is by far the more potent factor.

4. Alcoholic mental disease may result either from regular or from periodic drinking. Of the patients included in this study, nearly 70 per cent were regular drinkers.

5. A fixed habit of excessive drinking with frequent intoxication preceded the onset of mental disease in the great majority of the cases studied.

6. Reduction of efficiency in employment and loss of position commonly precede the onset of alcoholic mental disease.

7. Impairment of physical health frequently results from excessive drinking prior to the onset of the mental disease.

8. A history of delirium tremens was obtained in 23.5 per cent of the 1920-1923 group and in 29.4 per cent of the 1936-1937 group.

9. The use of drugs is not an important factor in the causation of alcoholic mental disease.

10. Alcohol was reported as the principal etiological factor in 633 of the 649 ascertained cases of the 1920-1923 group and in 1,535 of the 1,570 ascertained cases of the 1936-1937 group.

11. No striking differences are noted in the use and effect of alcohol in relation to the mental disease of the two groups studied. The smaller annual number of alcoholic first admissions in the years 1920-1923 probably was the direct result of a reduction in excessive drinking.

12. The data set forth in this chapter indicate that alcoholic mental disease is subject to control. The restriction placed on the sale of alcoholic beverages during the period 1920-1923, inclusive, caused a marked decline in alcoholism and its sequela, alcoholic mental disease. The failure in the enforcement of prohibition, and the liberal laws of 1933 and 1934 were followed by increases in alcoholic disorders. Some other more effective methods of control are clearly needed.

CHAPTER XV

Thirty Years of Alcoholic Mental Disease in New York State

The bureau of statistics of the State Hospital Commission and of its successor the State Department of Mental Hygiene has systematically compiled data concerning alcoholic mental disease since October 1, 1908. The civil State hospitals have sent to the statistical bureau at the end of each fiscal year a statistical schedule card for each first admission with alcoholic mental disease; also a card for each discharge, readmission or death of a patient with this class of disorder. The schedules have been uniform for all hospitals. The hospital physicians in making diagnoses and in supplying other data called for by the schedules have been guided by a statistical manual which was carefully prepared by a committee composed of representatives of the State hospitals and of the statistical bureau. With respect to alcoholic mental disease, the classification set forth in the manual has remained essentially the same during the 30 fiscal years from 1909 to 1938, inclusive, which are covered by this study.

The purpose of the study is to give a statistical review of alcoholic mental disease in the State as shown by the cases admitted and treated in civil State hospitals connected with the Department of Mental Hygiene. Naturally, it is hoped that the facts set forth will suggest ways for prevention of this form of mental disorder. The data presented do not include all the cases of alcoholic mental disease which occurred in the State during the period covered. The statistical bureau has no record of the patients who are treated in their own homes, or of those who receive temporary treatment in general hospitals, or of voluntary cases in licensed institutions. It is believed, however, that the cases of alcoholic mental disease treated by the civil State hospitals constitute by far the larger part of those occurring in the State.

The primary cause of alcoholic mental disease is overindulgence in alcoholic beverages for a period of years. A few drinkers break down early from the effects of excessive drinking, while others develop sufficient resistance to withstand the effects of overindulgence for a score of years or more.

It is sometimes claimed that the person who develops alcoholic mental disease is an abnormal individual who acquires the drink habit because of his abnormality, or perhaps because of mental conflicts from which he seeks relief. There can be no doubt that certain cases of alcoholic mental disease can be accounted for in this manner, but comprehensive statistical studies in this State and elsewhere tend to indicate that the great majority of persons who develop alcoholic mental disease are average citizens who show no marked abnormality prior to the formation of the alcohol habit.

TABLE 1. FIRST ADMISSIONS WITH ALCOHOLIC MENTAL DISEASE, 1909-1938

Year	Number			Per cent of all first admissions			Number per 100,000 of general population**		
	M.	F.	T.	M.	F.	T.	M.	F.	T.
1909	433	128	561	15.6	5.8	10.8	9.7	2.9	6.3
1910	452	131	583	15.3	5.0	10.5	9.9	2.9	6.4
1911	444	147	591	14.7	5.5	10.4	9.6	3.2	6.4
1912	434	131	565	14.4	4.8	9.8	9.3	2.8	6.1
1913	438	134	572	13.7	4.7	9.4	9.2	2.8	6.1
1914	348	116	464	10.4	3.6	7.4	7.3	2.4	4.9
1915	255	90	345	7.8	3.1	5.6	5.3	1.9	3.6
1916	*215	*82	*297	8.4	3.5	6.1	†5.9	†2.2	†4.1
1917	437	157	594	12.1	4.8	8.6	8.8	3.2	6.0
1918	257	97	354	7.3	3.0	5.2	5.1	1.9	3.5
1919	204	65	269	5.8	2.0	4.0	4.0	1.3	2.6
1920	90	32	122	2.7	1.0	1.9	1.7	0.6	1.2
1921	167	26	193	4.6	0.8	2.8	3.2	0.5	1.8
1922	194	32	226	5.1	1.0	3.2	3.6	0.6	2.1
1923	220	56	276	6.1	1.7	4.0	4.1	1.0	2.6
1924	302	71	373	8.2	2.2	5.4	5.5	1.3	3.4
1925	341	81	422	8.8	2.3	5.7	6.2	1.5	3.8
1926	333	89	422	8.4	2.7	5.8	5.9	1.6	3.7
1927	440	114	554	10.1	3.2	7.0	7.6	2.0	4.8
1928	430	79	509	9.1	2.0	5.9	7.2	1.3	4.3
1929	459	78	537	9.7	2.0	6.3	7.5	1.3	4.4
1930	446	100	546	9.0	2.4	6.0	7.1	1.6	4.4
1931	497	102	599	9.8	2.4	6.5	7.7	1.6	4.7
1932	462	131	593	8.3	2.9	5.8	7.0	2.0	4.5
1933	556	150	706	9.3	3.0	6.5	8.3	2.2	5.3
1934	724	160	884	11.6	3.1	7.8	10.5	2.3	6.5
1935	620	164	784	10.1	3.0	6.8	8.8	2.4	5.6
1936	638	188	826	10.0	3.4	6.9	8.9	2.6	5.8
1937	714	163	877	10.5	2.8	7.0	9.7	2.3	6.0
1938	679	152	831	10.1	2.6	6.6	9.1	2.1	5.6

*Includes nine months due to change in fiscal year.

**Population of State in intercensal years is estimated. †Estimated for 12 months.

First Admissions, 1909-1938

The number and sex of new cases of alcoholic mental disease admitted annually to the New York civil State hospitals during the 30 years from 1909 to 1938, inclusive, are shown in Table 1. The table shows also for each year the percentage constituted by the alcoholic cases among all admissions and the rate of the alcoholic cases per 100,000 of general population. The data are also shown graphically in Chart 1.

The data in Table 1 reveal striking variations in the yearly first admissions during the period under consideration. It is presumed that a like variation occurred in the extent of alcoholic indulgence in the several years. For these effects certain causes, which will later be explained, stand out prominently; other causes undoubtedly operated but were less discernible. Starting with 1909, we find a rate of first admissions with alcoholic mental disease per 100,000 of population among males of 9.7 and among females of 2.9. During the next two years only minor changes in rate occurred, but in the following three years a declining trend was in evidence. In 1914, the rate for males dropped to 7.3 and the rate for females to 2.4. In the succeeding year there was a further decline in rates to 5.3 and 1.9, respectively. It is generally believed that the lessened frequency in alcoholic mental disease from 1912 to 1915 was due to the spread of "dry" territory in the State by means of local option and to the active propaganda against alcoholism carried on during this period.

The fiscal year which ended September 30, 1914, saw the beginning of the first World War. The succeeding four years constituted a period of apprehension and anxiety. The rate of new alcoholic cases among males shot up from 5.3 in 1915 to 8.8 in 1917, and among females from 1.9 to 3.2.

Following the entrance of the United States into the war, April 6, 1917, a new era with respect to the liquor traffic was ushered in. To aid in the training of enlisted men, the sale of intoxicating liquors at any military station or cantonment, or to any member of the military forces while in uniform, was prohibited by an act of Congress approved May 18, 1917. To save food supplies, the distillation of alcoholic beverages from grains and other foodstuffs was prohibited September 8, 1917, for the duration of the

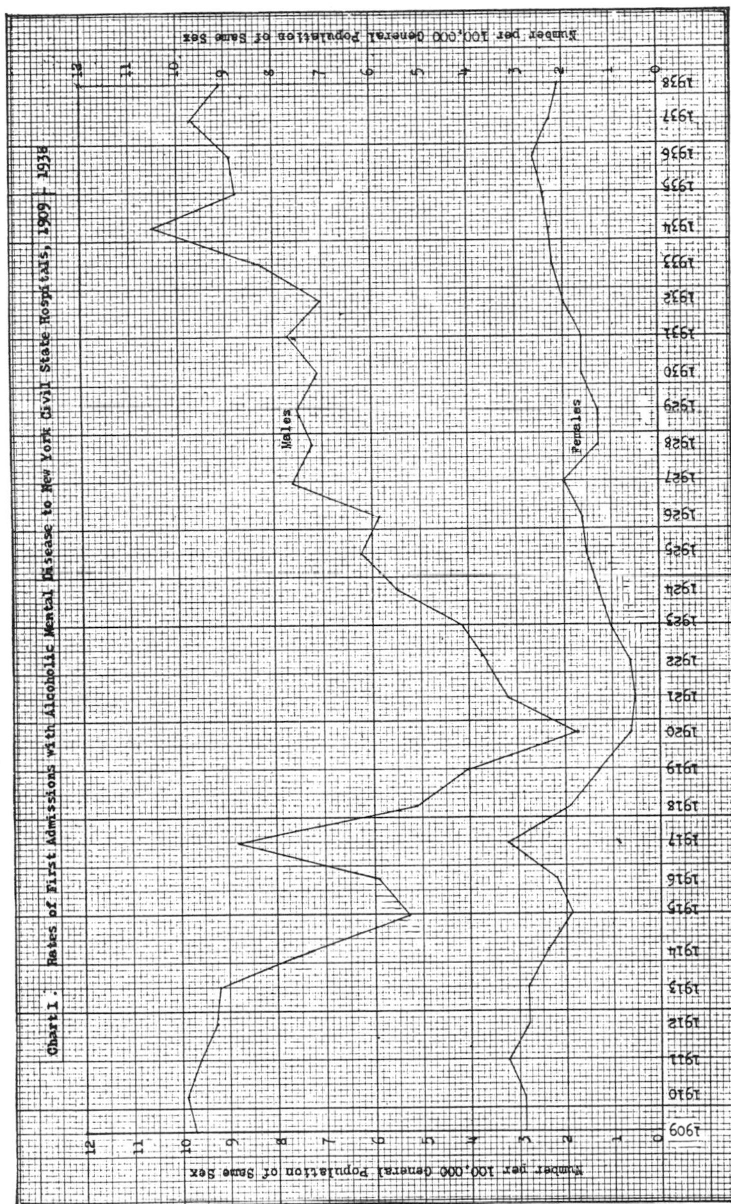

Chart I. Rates of First Admissions with Alcoholic Mental Disease to New York Civil State Hospitals, 1909 - 1938

war. Congress passed a resolution in December, 1917, submitting a prohibition amendment to the states. By January 16, 1919, this amendment had been ratified by three-fourths of the states. It went into effect January 17, 1920. Previous to the full ratification of the amendment, the President had signed (November 21, 1918) the Food Stimulation Bill providing for nationwide prohibition from June 30, 1919, until the demobilization of the army.

In New York State, similar restrictions were placed on the liquor traffic by acts of the State Legislature. Chapter 521 of the Laws of 1917 authorized the excise commissioner to suspend the sale of liquor in the proximity of camps or barracks for State or Federal troops, or near munition factories. In 1919, the State Legislature ratified the prohibition amendment. Chapter 155 of the Laws of 1921 amended Article 113 of the Penal Law, repealed the liquor tax law and the local option law, and prohibited the manufacture and sale of intoxicating liquor for beverage purposes. Chapter 5 of the Laws of 1921 required peace officers to enforce the provisions of Article 113 of the Penal Law relating to intoxicating liquors.

The effect of these restrictive measures, together with the elevation of the national morale, which had occurred during the war, is seen in the marked decline in new cases of alcoholic mental disease admitted to the civil State hospitals from 1917 to 1922. In the former year, 594 cases had been admitted; in 1920 the number dropped to the low point of 122 and was only 193 in 1921 and 226 in 1922. In other states, similar reduction in alcoholic admissions was reported. In Massachusetts, for example, the new alcoholic cases declined from 511 in 1917 to 102 in 1920.

In spite of the overwhelming sentiment supporting the restrictions placed on the liquor traffic during the war, a large minority was ready to criticize the operations of the prohibitory laws when peace was restored. Individual criticisms were succeeded by organized propaganda and organized violations. Opponents of the laws obtained political support and in New York State in 1923 were able to secure repeal, by Chapter 871 of the Laws of 1923, of Article 113 of the Penal Law and Section 802b of the Code of Criminal Procedure which provided for the enforcement of State laws relating to the liquor traffic.

In the absence of State control, violators multiplied; the over-indulgence in alcoholic beverages which followed is reflected in the increased number of alcoholic first admissions occurring from 1923 to 1927. The new cases in the latter year numbered 554, the largest number in any one year since 1917. The trend in alcoholic admissions was almost level during the succeeding five years.

In 1933 came the repeal of the Eighteenth Amendment and the passage in New York State of the Alcoholic Beverage Control Law, Chapter 180 of the Laws of 1933. This law was superseded by Chapter 474 of the Laws of 1934. The first law placed the supervision of the liquor traffic in an "Alcoholic Beverage Control Board"; the second law designated the board as "The State Liquor Authority". This authority consists of five members. The New York City Alcoholic Beverage Control Board has four members, and county boards each have two members. The State Liquor Authority is given power to issue and revoke licenses for the sale of intoxicating liquors, but the enforcement of the law devolves on local officials. Under this law the liquor traffic probably has more liberty than at any time subsequent to 1896, when the original State Liquor Tax Law was enacted (Chapter 112, Laws of 1896).

The institution of the new laws in 1933 and 1934 was accompanied by a marked upward rise in the admissions of new cases of alcoholic mental disease. The number increased from 593 in 1932 to 706 in 1933, and to 884 in 1934. The substantial reduction which occurred in 1935 was followed by increases which were not as marked as those of 1933 and 1934.

Chart 1 shows clearly the extent by which male admissions with alcoholic disease exceed the female. The fluctuations in rates among men, thought to be due principally to changes in legal restrictions on the liquor traffic, are striking. It is believed that the trends in alcoholic first admissions as shown by Chart 1 constitute a rough index of the consumption of alcoholic beverages. As consumption increases, alcoholic admissions to mental hospitals increase.* Convictions for intoxication are likewise affected.

*Pollock, H. M.: Alcoholic psychoses before and after prohibition. Ment. Hyg., VI:4, October, 1922.

Further light is shown on the origin of the alcoholic cases by Table 2 and Chart 2. It is evident that the cases come principally from cities and it is noteworthy that female cases in cities are more numerous than male cases in rural districts. The fluctuations in rates above described are seen to be due mainly to the variations

TABLE 2. FIRST ADMISSIONS WITH ALCOHOLIC MENTAL DISEASE TO NEW YORK CIVIL STATE HOSPITALS, (classified according to environment), 1909-1938

Year	Total			Urban			Rural†			Unascertained and other states		
	M.	F.	T.	M.	F.	T.	M.	F.	T.	M.	F.	T.
1909	433	128	561	356	115	471	69	11	80	8	2	10
1910	452	131	583	361	121	482	87	8	95	4	2	6
1911	444	147	591	406	142	548	34	4	38	4	1	5
1912	434	131	565	353	121	474	75	8	83	6	2	8
1913	438	134	572	387	129	516	47	4	51	4	1	5
1914	348	116	464	316	115	431	31	1	32	1	..	1
1915	255	90	345	194	81	275	61	9	70	..	..	..
1916*	215	82	297	195	80	275	20	2	22	..	..	..
1917	437	157	594	389	148	537	45	7	52	3	2	5
1918	257	97	354	215	94	309	41	3	44	1	..	1
1919	204	65	269	180	63	243	24	2	26	..	..	..
1920	90	32	122	80	30	110	10	1	11	..	1	1
1921	167	26	193	156	26	182	11	..	11	..	..	..
1922	194	32	226	177	32	209	15	..	15	2	..	2
1923	220	56	276	205	53	258	15	3	18	..	..	..
1924	302	71	373	271	71	342	31	..	31	..	..	..
1925	341	81	422	308	78	386	33	3	36	..	..	..
1926	333	89	422	293	85	378	39	4	43	1	..	1
1927	440	114	554	395	111	506	41	3	44	4	..	4
1928	430	79	509	392	76	468	37	3	40	1	..	1
1929	459	78	537	407	75	482	52	3	55	..	..	..
1930	446	100	546	418	98	516	28	2	30	..	..	..
1931	497	102	599	443	97	540	54	5	59	..	..	..
1932	462	131	593	421	128	549	40	3	43	1	..	1
1933	556	150	706	498	147	645	41	2	43	17	1	18
1934	724	160	884	662	152	814	47	7	54	15	1	16
1935	620	164	784	554	160	714	53	4	57	13	..	13
1936	638	188	826	566	179	745	56	6	62	16	3	19
1937	714	163	877	644	154	798	57	6	63	13	3	16
1938	679	152	831	613	142	755	56	8	64	10	2	12
Total	12,229	3,246	15,475	10,855	3,103	13,958	1,250	122	1,372	124	21	145

*Includes nine months due to change in fiscal year.

†Includes villages from 1909-1915.

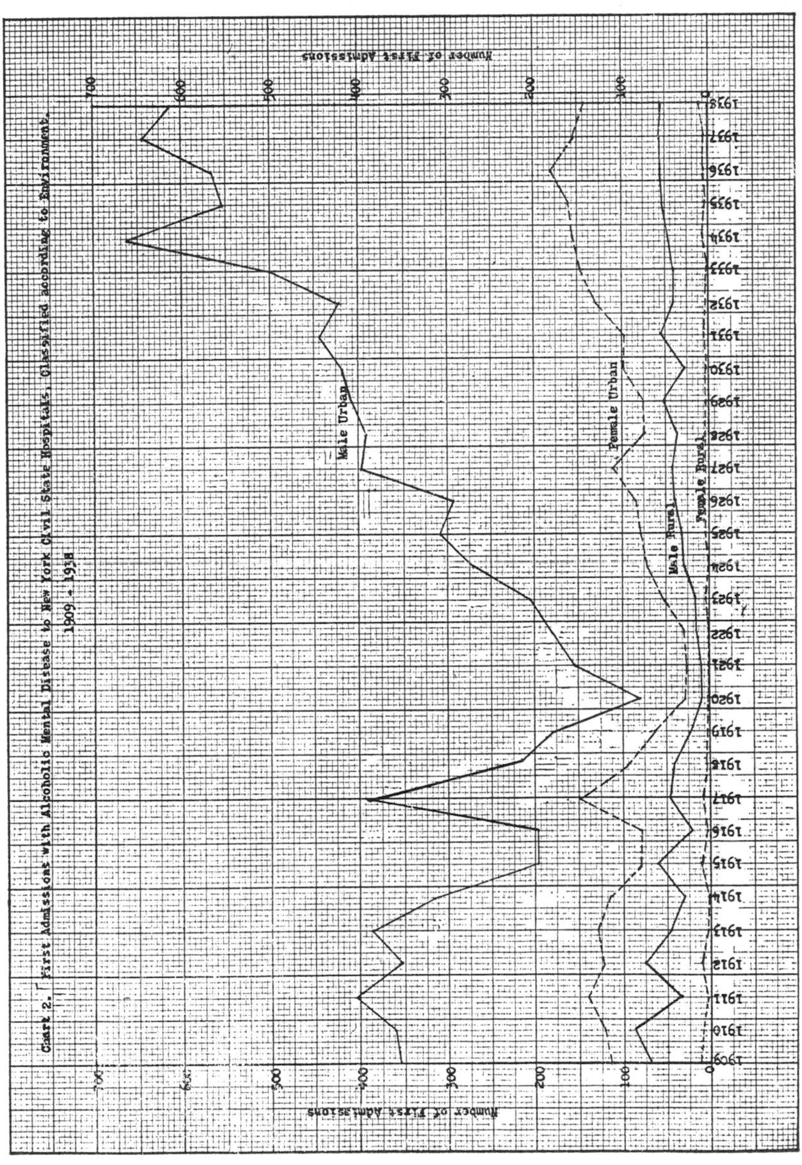
Chart 2. First Admissions with Alcoholic Mental Disease to New York Civil State Hospitals, Classified according to Environment.
1909 - 1938
Number of First Admissions
700
600
500
400
300
200
100
0
Male Urban
Female Urban
Male Rural
Female Rural
1909
1910
1911
1912
1913
1914
1915
1916
1917
1918
1919
1920
1921
1922
1923
1924
1925
1926
1927
1928
1929
1930
1931
1932
1933
1934
1935
1936
1937
1938

in male urban admissions. Only 122 female cases were admitted from rural districts during the entire 30 years covered by the study. In 1921, 1922 and 1924 there were no female cases from rural districts. Apparently, changes in legal restrictions are reflected to the greatest extent by male admissions from cities.

The race distribution of the alcoholic first admissions is shown for the years 1914 to 1938 in Table 3. Of the 12,603 admissions,

TABLE 3. RACIAL DISTRIBUTION, FIRST ADMISSIONS WITH ALCOHOLIC MENTAL DISEASE TO NEW YORK CIVIL STATE HOSPITALS, 1914-1938

Year	Total			White		Negro		All other races	
	M.	F.	T.	M.	F.	M.	F.	M.	F.
1914	348	116	464	342	112	6	4	..	..
1915	255	90	345	248	89	7	1	..	..
1916* ...	215	82	297	206	80	9	2	..	..
1917	437	157	594	423	149	14	8	..	..
1918	257	97	354	248	92	9	5	..	..
1919	204	65	269	196	63	8	2	..	..
1920	90	32	122	89	31	1	1	..	..
1921	167	26	193	157	25	5	1	5	..
1922	194	32	226	190	30	4	2	..	..
1923	220	56	276	213	54	5	2	2	..
1924	302	71	373	279	66	23	5	..	..
1925	341	81	422	329	78	11	3	1	..
1926	333	89	422	319	85	12	4	2	..
1927	440	114	554	407	98	30	16	3	..
1928	430	79	509	402	70	23	8	5	1
1929	459	78	537	415	64	34	13	10	1
1930	446	100	546	393	86	43	14	10	..
1931	497	102	599	452	81	39	20	6	1
1932	462	131	593	411	114	48	14	3	3
1933	556	150	706	501	124	54	26	1	..
1934	724	160	884	627	122	94	38	3	..
1935	620	164	784	523	126	94	38	3	..
1936	638	188	826	535	145	100	43	3	..
1937	714	163	877	593	125	117	38	4	..
1938	679	152	831	581	113	97	39	1	..
Total	10,028	2,575	12,603	9,079	2,222	887	347	62	6

*Includes nine months due to change in fiscal year.

11,301, or 89.7 per cent, were white; 1,234, or 9.8, were negroes; and 68, or 0.5, were members of other races. A surprisingly small number of negroes was admitted prior to 1924. Before that year, the annual number of negro males admitted exceeded 10 only in 1917 and the number of negro females did not exceed 10 in any year prior to 1927.

On account of the small number of negro first admissions and the rapid changes in the negro general population, satisfactory comparative rates for whites and negroes for the several years cannot be computed. In the year 1920, only two negro alcoholic cases were admitted. In the year of 1930, the rate per 100,000 of general population of same race for the negroes was 13.8 and for the whites, 3.94. From 1933 to 1938 noteworthy increases in negro admissions occurred.

Outcome of Alcoholic Mental Disease

Table 4 shows discharges and deaths along with first admissions and readmissions of patients with alcoholic mental disease for each year from 1909 to 1938. In the entire period there were 15,475 first admissions, 3,104 readmissions, 13,239 discharges, and 3,633 deaths in the hospitals. The number of readmissions was 20.1 per cent of the number of first admissions and 23.4 per cent of the number of discharges. The number of patients dying in the hospitals was 23.5 per cent of the number of first admissions.

The annual recovery rates by sex per 100 of all admissions are shown in Table 5 and Chart 3. These rates fluctuate to a marked extent because of variations in both admissions and recoveries. As a rule in this mental disorder, recovery rates are higher among males than among females. It is probable that some of the latter are admitted in a late stage of the disease from which recovery is difficult. The general recovery rate for the males for the entire period was 53.4, and for the females, 42.7.

TABLE 4. ADMISSIONS, DISCHARGES AND DEATHS OF PATIENTS WITH ALCOHOLIC MENTAL DISEASE, NEW YORK CIVIL STATE HOSPITALS, 1909-1938

Year	Admissions				Discharges						Deaths in hospital	
	First		Readmissions		Recovered		Much improved and improved		Unimproved			
	M.	F.	M.	F.	M.	F.	M.	F.	M.	F.	M.	F.
1909 ..	433	128	93	17	258	70	78	14	12	5	61	28
1910 ..	452	131	94	17	323	65	83	19	14	2	86	33
1911 ..	444	147	86	26	288	60	97	29	16	3	80	37
1912 ..	434	131	95	22	288	71	100	25	23	3	87	43
1913 ..	438	134	97	21	275	61	103	29	27	3	80	31
1914 ..	348	116	70	21	269	55	96	41	23	1	89	45
1915 ..	255	90	66	21	178	46	91	34	9	2	69	37
1916* .	215	82	40	16	104	29	43	25	5	3	54	36
1917 ..	437	157	73	17	220	49	68	32	2	3	97	50
1918 ..	257	97	54	16	195	43	80	44	2	1	94	36
1919 ..	204	65	43	10	149	33	78	40	3	4	79	32
1920 ..	90	32	27	5	115	29	44	20	4	2	55	23
1921 ..	167	26	37	5	99	19	45	16	10	..	54	26
1922 ..	194	32	35	11	128	15	51	14	6	1	47	24
1923 ..	220	56	45	15	148	30	39	9	6	..	52	30
1924 ..	302	71	53	21	196	28	45	25	11	3	62	29
1925 ..	341	81	67	13	211	40	56	14	9	3	72	41
1926 ..	333	89	69	17	236	42	55	24	11	2	91	53
1927 ..	440	114	64	14	261	47	59	14	10	3	78	48
1928 ..	430	79	73	14	254	51	77	10	12	1	79	28
1929 ..	459	78	76	19	224	40	93	13	5	1	97	36
1930 ..	446	100	78	16	304	48	94	19	12	1	78	30
1931 ..	497	102	88	15	285	57	103	18	10	1	114	42
1932 ..	462	131	84	18	315	55	75	19	8	1	116	28
1933 ..	556	150	98	25	301	85	78	23	13	2	93	34
1934 ..	724	160	127	29	397	83	116	29	12	3	122	42
1935 ..	620	164	152	30	491	92	143	26	16	1	125	36
1936 ..	638	188	153	36	443	93	150	41	9	6	123	39
1937 ..	714	163	186	36	450	93	150	47	12	1	125	45
1938 ..	679	152	203	35	474	104	188	49	9	4	93	39
Total	12,229	3,246	2,526	578	7,879	1,633	2,578	762	321	66	2,552	1,081

*Includes nine months due to change in fiscal year.

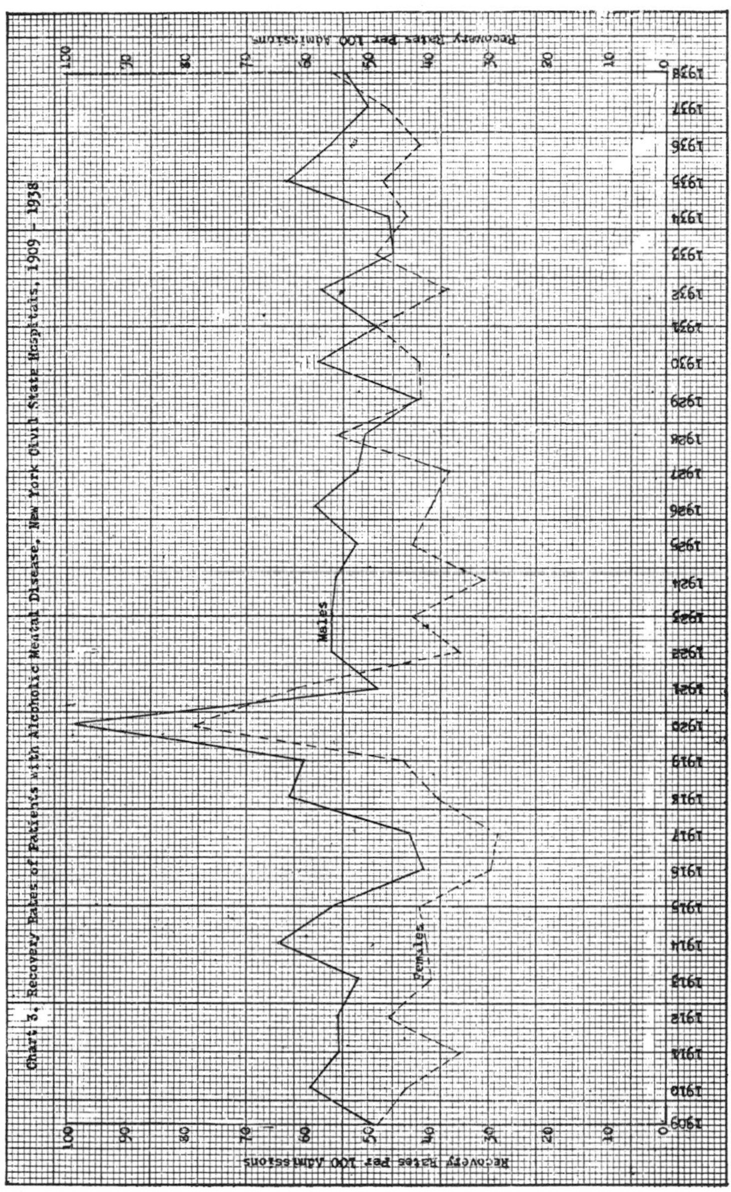

Chart 3. Recovery Rates of Patients with Alcoholic Mental Disease, New York Civil State Hospitals, 1909 - 1938

TABLE 5. RECOVERY RATES PER 100 ADMISSIONS OF PATIENTS WITH ALCOHOLIC MENTAL DISEASE, NEW YORK CIVIL STATE HOSPITALS, 1909-1938

Year	Males	Females	Total
1909	49.0	48.3	48.9
1910	59.2	43.9	55.9
1911	54.3	34.7	49.5
1912	54.4	46.4	52.6
1913	51.4	39.4	48.7
1914	64.4	40.1	58.4
1915	55.5	41.4	51.9
1916*	40.8	29.6	37.7
1917	43.1	28.2	39.3
1918	62.7	38.1	56.1
1919	60.3	44.0	56.5
1920	98.3	78.4	93.5
1921	48.5	61.3	50.2
1922	55.9	34.9	52.6
1923	55.8	42.3	53.0
1924	55.2	30.4	50.1
1925	51.7	42.6	50.0
1926	58.7	39.6	54.7
1927	51.8	36.7	48.7
1928	50.5	54.8	51.2
1929	41.9	41.2	41.8
1930	58.0	41.4	55.0
1931	48.7	48.7	48.7
1932	57.7	36.9	53.2
1933	46.0	48.6	46.6
1934	46.7	43.9	46.2
1935	63.6	47.4	60.4
1936	56.0	41.5	52.8
1937	50.0	46.7	49.4
1938	53.7	55.6	54.1

*Includes nine months due to change in fiscal year.

In Chart 3, the fluctuations in recovery rates follow a jagged sawtooth pattern except in the years 1918 to 1922 when exceptionally high rates are seen for both males and females. The reduction in admissions in 1919, 1920 and 1921 was undoubtedly a factor in the causation of the high recovery rates in those years.

Annual death rates per 1,000 patients with alcoholic mental disease under treatment are available only for the years from 1917 to 1938. The rates for the several years are shown in Table 6 and

TABLE 6. DEATH RATES PER 1,000 UNDER TREATMENT OF PATIENTS WITH ALCOHOLIC MENTAL DISEASE, NEW YORK CIVIL STATE HOSPITALS, 1917-1938

Year	Males	Females	Total
1917	60.6	70.6	63.7
1918	60.0	53.9	58.2
1919	54.4	52.4	53.8
1920	44.0	42.5	43.6
1921	44.4	50.9	46.3
1922	37.5	49.1	40.7
1923	40.4	59.9	45.9
1924	43.6	54.8	46.7
1925	47.8	76.8	55.4
1926	58.1	97.8	68.3
1927	46.0	88.2	56.3
1928	44.2	53.6	46.3
1929	51.3	67.2	54.8
1930	40.2	54.1	43.3
1931	55.8	74.7	59.9
1932	56.3	48.5	54.6
1933	42.9	52.1	45.1
1934	48.8	61.4	51.5
1935	47.7	50.3	48.3
1936	46.9	49.7	47.5
1937	45.2	56.0	47.7
1938	32.5	48.8	36.1

Chart 4. The rate for both sexes combined varies from 36.1 in 1938 to 68.3 in 1926. The rate for males varies from 32.5 in 1938 to 60.6 in 1917; and the rate for females from 42.5 in 1920 to 97.8 in 1926. The striking fluctuations in rates are seen at a glance in Chart 4. The generally higher death rates among females may indicate that the disease affects females more seriously or that the female patients are in poorer condition when admitted. The latter is probably the more plausible explanation.

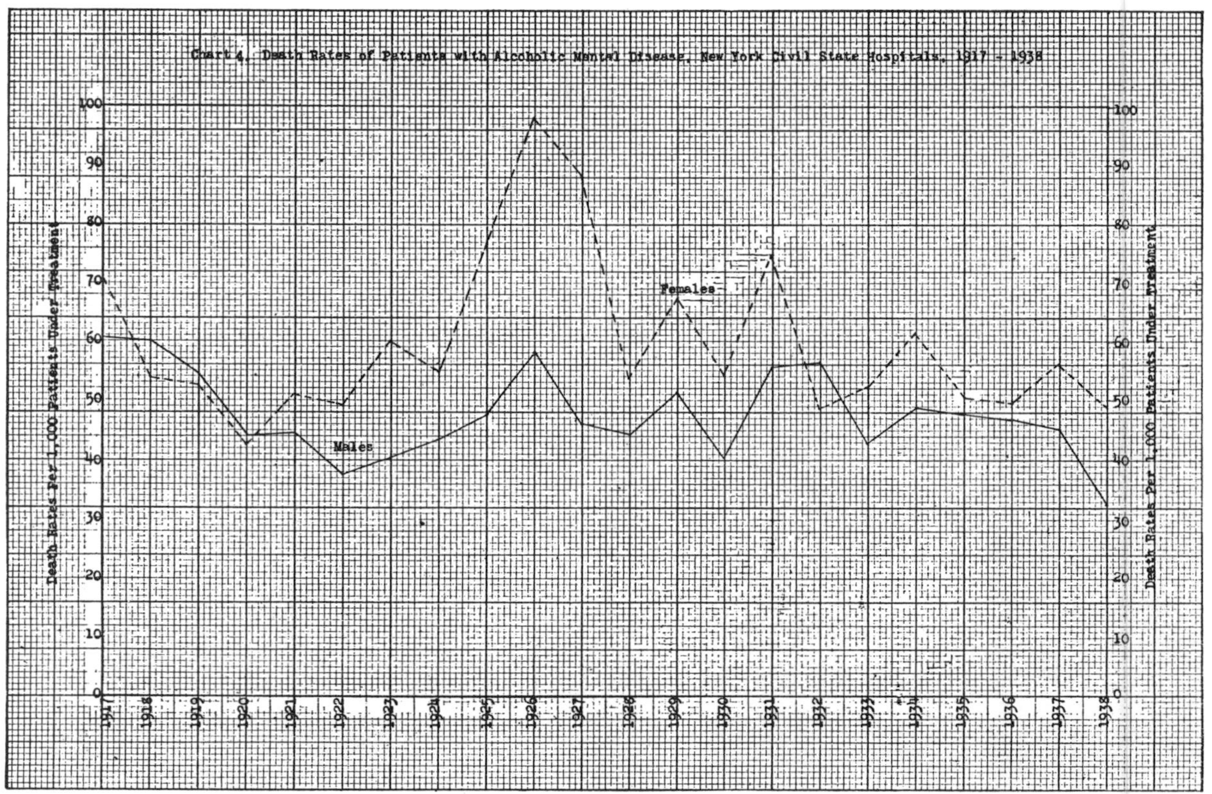
Chart 4. Death Rates of Patients with Alcoholic Mental Disease, New York Civil State Hospitals, 1917 - 1938
Death Rates Per 1,000 Patients Under Treatment
100
90
80
70
60
50
40
30
20
10
0
1917
1918
1919
1920
1921
1922
1923
1924
1925
1926
1927
1928
1929
1930
1931
1932
1933
1934
1935
1936
1937
1938
Females
Males
Death Rates Per 1,000 Patients Under Treatment

Reference to Chart 4 shows that comparatively low death rates prevailed in both sexes from 1919 to 1922. The rates rapidly increased in succeeding years, especially among females, and reached their high point in 1926. Then followed a rapid decline for two years and marked irregularity for the succeeding nine years. Low rates for both males and females occurred in 1938.

Alcoholic Admissions to Bellevue Hospital

An interesting sidelight on the effects of the consumption of alcoholic beverages during the 30 years under review is found in the accompanying table (No. 7) which was furnished the writer by

Table 7. Alcoholic Admissions to Bellevue Hospital*

Year	Male	Female	Total
1909	8,086	2,435	10,521
1910	8,610	2,697	11,307
1911	7,111	2,427	9,538
1912	6,459	2,278	8,737
1913	6,609	2,131	8,740
1914	6,394	2,234	8,628
1915	6,014	2,063	8,077
1916	6,829	2,092	8,921
1917	5,076	1,367	6,443
1918	4,525	3,260	7,785
1919	4,810	3,152	7,962
1920	1,642	449	2,091
1921	1,931	450	2,381
1922	3,305	778	4,083
1923	4,685	1,092	5,777
1924	5,295	1,139	6,434
1925	4,880	1,055	5,935
1926	4,938	986	5,924
1927	5,520	1,027	6,547
1928	5,881	1,118	6,999
1929	5,995	1,071	7,066
1930	7,337	1,432	8,769
1931	8,037	1,331	9,368
1932	7,049	1,212	8,261
1933	8,260	1,282	9,542
1934	6,279	1,370	7,649
1935	7,506	1,633	9,139
1936	10,064	1,892	11,956
1937	9,532	1,861	11,393
1938	9,953	2,131	12,084

*Includes inebriates and patients with alcoholic mental disease.

Dr. Norman Jolliffe of Bellevue Hospital, New York City. The table shows the alcoholic admissions to that hospital during the 30 years, 1909 to 1938, inclusive. Such admissions consist in part of inebriates and in part of persons suffering from alcoholic mental disease. Many of the cases are picked up by the police on the streets of the city and sent to Bellevue Hospital for examination and treatment.

Referring to Table 7, we note that in 1909 there were 10,521 alcoholic admissions to the Bellevue Hospital. In the succeeding year the admissions increased to 11,307. This figure was not exceeded until 1936. Beginning with 1911, a declining trend in admissions set in. With some irregularity the decline continued to 1920, when only 2,091 alcoholic cases were admitted. In 1921, the number increased slightly to 2,381. A marked upward trend began in 1922, when the admissions increased to 4,083. The rising trend continued with slight interruptions to 1938. In that year the number of alcoholic admissions was 12,084—the largest annual number in the entire period of 30 years. The trends in the admissions of males and females are in general similar but have some peculiar divergencies. The increase in female admissions from 1,367 in 1917 to 3,260 in 1918 is unexplainable. A similar jump in male admissions from 7,506 in 1935 to 10,064 in 1936 occurred without apparent adequate cause.

The frequency of the admissions to Bellevue during the 30 years covered by this study corresponds in general with the frequency of the cases of alcoholic mental disease admitted to the civil State hospitals as shown in previous tables. This fact indicates that the influences affecting the use of liquors during this period were operative not only in bringing patients to mental hospitals in varying numbers, but also in causing fluctuations in cases of inebriety. New York City, however, was not affected by local option. As previously mentioned, in the rural districts of the State there was considerable "dry" territory before the days of prohibtion and the increase of such territory undoubtedly affected the rate of alcoholic admissions to mental hospitals. However, anti-alcoholic propaganda appears to have had considerable effect in New York City, as the rate of admissions declined previous to wartime restrictions on the liquor traffic.

Comment

In view of the fact that alcoholic mental disease is preventable and that effective methods for its prevention are known and are available, the data submitted in the foregoing review should have more than academic interest. In the 30 years reviewed, 15,475 persons in this State developed mental disease attributable to overindulgence in alcoholic liquors and were admitted to the civil State hospitals. During the three years 1936, 1937 and 1938, the new alcoholic admissions averaged 843 per year. Although a large part of these patients will be discharged after treatment, they are likely to resume their former drinking habits. To a considerable degree, they represent a social and economic loss to society.

Table 7 shows that in the years 1936, 1937 and 1938 a total of 35,433 patients were admitted to the Bellevue Hospital for inebriety and alcoholic mental disease. The yearly average was 11,811. It is probable that most of these individuals have a confirmed alcoholic habit. According to reports of the Department of Correction, the total convictions in courts of special sessions for intoxication in New York State in the three years above mentioned were 112,609, an average of 37,536 per year. It may safely be assumed that such number represents but a small fraction of the persons who became intoxicated during a year.

These official figures show clearly the need of effectual measures for the prevention of alcoholism and alcoholic mental disease.

Thus far, most preventive measures have been directed toward the restriction of the liquor traffic. During the war period from 1914 to 1919 and for a few years thereafter, such measures produced the desired results. Later, sentiment in favor of the enforcement of restrictive laws died down, hence the laws became unpopular and noneffective.

For many years previous to prohibition, school children in New York State were taught the effects of alcoholic beverages and other narcotics. During and following prohibition, such teaching ceased to be emphasized.

The present Alcoholic Beverage Control Law prohibits the sale of alcoholic beverages to minors under 18 years of age, to intoxicated persons and to habitual drunkards. No provision is made for the effectual enforcement of these provisions. The extent of their violation may be estimated from data concerning intoxication, alcoholism and alcoholic mental disease set forth in this article. It is evident that an alcoholic beverage control law which provides for licensing by a state board and for enforcement by local officials is virtually noneffective in preventing intoxication and other effects of overindulgence in alcoholic liquors.

A scientific approach to the problem is needed. The economic, political, social and health aspects should receive the most careful study. If it is found that the taxes paid by the liquor traffic are not largely extracted from the earnings of the poor; if it is found that the drink habit makes workers in all occupations more reliable and more efficient; if it is found that the free use of alcoholic beverages promotes health and good citizenship and lessens crime and accidents; if it is found that the liquor traffic as a whole constitutes a real asset in the balance sheet of human welfare—if these things are found, then the liquor traffic should be encouraged, and everyone, both young and old, should form the drink habit. If the findings of the study do not reveal the benefits mentioned but the opposite, appropriate action should be taken. The effectual measures taken by health departments to control communicable disease might receive consideration. Relief from intoxication, alcoholism and alcoholic mental disease cannot be obtained by collecting fees, closing the eyes and saying "All is well".

BIBLIOGRAPHY

Brown, Frederick W.: Alcoholic mental disease before and after prohibition. Read before annual meeting of the American Statistical Association, Washington, D. C., December 30, 1931.

Emerson, Haven: Alcohol and Man. The Macmillan Company, New York, 1932.

Graham, Whidden: Alcoholic beverages and insanity. N. Am. Rev., April, 1918.

Guthrie, Riley H., and Dayton, Neil A.: The incidence of alcoholic psychoses in Massachusetts, 1917-1935. N. E. Jour. Med. 216:5.

Jolliffe, Norman: The alcoholic admissions to Bellevue Hospital. Sci., 83:2152, March 27, 1936.

Miles, Walter R.: Psychological factors in alcoholism. Ment. Hyg., XXI:4, October, 1937.

Pollock, Horatio M.: A statistical study of 1,739 patients with alcoholic psychoses. State Hosp. Bul., August, 1914.

——: The use and effect of alcohol in relation to the alcoholic psychoses. State Hosp. Bul., August, 1915.

——: Decline of alcohol as a cause of insanity. Psychiat. Bul., April, 1917.

——: Decline of alcohol and drugs as causes of mental disease. Ment. Hyg., V:1, January, 1921.

——: Alcoholic psychoses before and after prohibition. Ment. Hyg., VI:4, October, 1922.

——: Prohibition and alcoholic mental disease. Ment. Hyg., VIII:2, April, 1924. (With Edith M. Furbush.)

——: Recent statistics of alcoholic mental disease. Ment. Hyg., XIII:3, July, 1929. (With Frederick W. Brown.)

——: The prevalence of mental disease due to alcoholism. (In: Alcohol and Man. Haven Emerson, M. D., editor, q. v., pp. 344-372.)

——: Use and effect of alcohol in relation to alcoholic mental disease before, during, and after prohibition. Ment. Hyg., XXIV:1, January, 1940.

Wall, James Hardin: A study of alcoholism in men. Am. Jour. Psychiat., 92:6, May, 1936.

——: A study of alcoholism in women. Am. Jour. Psychiat., 93:4, January, 1937.

Williams, Frankwood E.: The relation of alcohol and syphilis to mental hygiene. Am. Jour. Pub. Health, 6:12.

Alcohol Beverage Control Law, Chapter 478 of New York State Laws, 1934.

Liquor Tax Law of the State of New York. Chapter 39 of the Laws of 1909, and amendments.

CHAPTER XVI

Is the Paroled Patient a Menace to the Community?*

The charge is frequently made that the paroling of mental patients by State hospitals is a dangerous procedure. If a patient commits an offense while on parole, the sensational press gives the incident wide publicity and endeavors to make the public believe that every paroled patient is a menace to the community. Influenced by the agitation of the matter, one of the New York legislators introduced a bill during the 1938 session of the State Legislature to establish special boards for the supervision of paroled patients in various parts of the State.

In order to ascertain the facts relative to the antisocial behavior of paroled patients, the State Department of Mental Hygiene instituted in February, 1938, an inquiry concerning the offenses committed by patients paroled from its State hospitals during the fiscal year ended June 30, 1937.

The New York State hospital system for mental patients comprises 18 large State hospitals in addition to a psychiatric institute and hospital and a psychopathic hospital. Of the 71,281 patients on the books of these hospitals on June 30, 1937, 64,767 were resident patients, 377 patients were in family care and 6,137 were on parole. In accordance with the policy of the department, patients who are considered eligible to leave the hospital are paroled for one year previous to being discharged. That the parole service is active is seen by the following tabulation:

Data Concerning Paroled Patients, New York Civil State Hospitals, 1937

	Males	Females	Total
Patients placed on parole during year	5,092	4,471	9,563
Patients returned from parole during year	2,249	1,645	3,894
Patients discharged from parole during year	2,415	2,273	4,688
Average number of patients on parole during year	2,951	2,882	5,833

Altogether the outpatient departments of the hospitals dealt with more than 14,000 patients during the year. The average daily number on parole was 5,833.

*Published in the Psychiatric Quarterly for April, 1938.

The offenses committed by paroled patients were as follows: By male patients: 26 misdemeanors and 11 felonies; by female patients: 3 misdemeanors and no felonies.

Based on average daily population the rate of misdemeanors per 1,000 paroled men was 8.8 and the rate of felonies, 3.7. The rate of misdemeanors among paroled women was 1.03 per 1,000. The rate of all offenses for both sexes combined was 6.9.

The foregoing rates are very small compared to rates of crime for the general population as reported by the New York State Department of Correction for the year 1937. According to such report the total number of crimes reported in the State in 1937 was 1,000,078. The rate per 1,000 of general population was 74.3. If the rate is computed on the basis of the population of the State 15 years of age and over, it becomes 98.5. From these data it appears that the rate of crime among the general population 15 years of age and over is about 14 times as high as that among paroled patients.

In the report of the Department of Correction, crimes are not classified by sex of persons committing them. Data concerning arrests, however, are shown by sex. Of the 1,012,524 persons arrested in the State during the year, 936,036 were men and 76,488 women. The rate of arrests per 1,000 of general population 15 years of age and over was 184.4 among men, 15.1 among women, and 99.7 among both sexes combined. The corresponding rates of arrests of paroled patients were 12.5 for the men, 1.03 for the women and 6.9 for both sexes combined. Bringing these data together we find that the rate of arrests among the so-called normal adult population as compared with the rate of arrests among paroled patients appears as follows:

COMPARISON OF ARRESTS AMONG GENERAL NORMAL ADULT POPULATION AND AMONG PAROLED PATIENTS, NEW YORK STATE, 1937

	General adult population			Paroled patients		
	Males	Females	Total	Males	Females	Total
Number of arrests	936,036	76,488	1,012,524	37	3	40
Rates of arrests per 1,000...	184.4	15.1	99.7	12.5	1.03	6.9

It will be observed that the rate of arrests among the general adult population for both sexes was over fourteen times as high as that among the paroled patients. In other words, in 1937, while 40 arrests were being made among this group of paroled patients approximately 576 arrests were being made among an average normal group of like size of the general population.

CLASSIFICATION OF OFFENSES COMMITTED BY PAROLED PATIENTS FROM NEW YORK CIVIL STATE HOSPITALS, 1937

	Males	Females	Total
Misdemeanors:			
Assault	2	..	2
Threatened assault	1	..	1
Disorderly conduct	7	1	8
Intoxication	6	2	8
Petit larceny	5	..	5
Reckless driving	1	..	1
Vagrancy	3	..	3
Unclassified	1	..	1
Total misdemeanors	26	3	29
Felonies:			
Assault	3	..	3
Forgery	3	..	3
Homicide	1	..	1
Larceny	1	..	1
Selling narcotics	2	..	2
Unlawful entry	1	..	1
Total felonies	11	..	11
Grand total	37	3	40

The accompanying table giving the classification of the offenses committed by paroled patients shows that 19 of the 29 misdemeanors were classed as disorderly conduct, intoxication and vagrancy. These minor offenses resulted in no serious harm to anyone. Among the felonies were one homicide and five assaults with dangerous weapons. The latter assaults as well as those classed as misdemeanors did not result in serious injuries. One of the forgeries reported was committed by an escaped convict who was a malingerer. He was brought to the State hospital feigning amnesia. Later he admitted he was shamming. He escaped from the hospital and, after 24 hours, was automatically placed on parole. He was subsequently arrested and convicted of forgery and housebreaking and sentenced to State prison.

The history of the patient who committed the only homicide reported is given by the State hospital, as follows:

"The patient, a male, 45 years of age, was admitted to the State hospital, September 3, 1936, having had a long history of alcoholism and irresponsibility, but without criminalistic tendencies. He quickly recovered from a typical attack of delirium tremens, was paroled November 4, 1936, and returned from parole November 13, 1936, after a renewal of alcoholic indulgence. At his aunt's urgent request and in the absence of psychotic symptoms, he was paroled again, November 25, 1936. The patient was seen by the social worker and by the hospital psychiatrists on a number of occasions, and his hospitalization in a general hospital or his return to the State hospital should any mental symptoms develop was urged several times, last on June 15, 1937. His aged aunts, who had overindulged him for many years, refused to return him to this hospital, but had sent him to a general hospital on one occasion. Periodically, he received treatment from a local physician, and on June 14, 1937, the Veterans' Relief Bureau promised hospitalization in a veterans' hospital should it be indicated. On June 28, 1937, in an intoxicated state, he attacked his two aunts with an axe, killing one and injuring the other so that she died shortly. Later, he pleaded guilty to second degree murder and was sentenced to Dannemora prison."

In this case the crime was clearly due to alcoholism and not to mental disease.

The findings of this inquiry showing a low rate of criminal offenses among paroled patients are supported by those of a study made in 1922 by Dr. Maurice C. Ashley, concerning the "Outcome of 1,000 Cases Paroled from Middletown State Homeopathic Hospital." The 1,000 cases were under observation on the average nearly five years. During this period 12 of the patients were arrested for various offenses including assault, vagrancy, forgery and swindlery. The average annual rate of arrests among the group was approximately 2.4 per 1,000. This rate is even lower than that found for the group that constitute the basis of the present study.

Further evidence of low rates of offenses among paroled and discharged patients is obtained from a study of posthospital histories of 741 patients paroled and discharged from Binghamton and Hudson River State hospitals. These histories covered a period of 10 years following the parole of the patients. They were prepared in 1930 and 1931 by field agents employed by the State Charities Aid Association under the direction of Mr. Raymond G. Fuller. The histories show that among the 289 male patients there were 19 arrests and among the 452 female patients 5 arrests. The annual rate of arrests among males was 0.7 per cent and among females 0.1 per cent.

The low rate of antisocial behavior among paroled patients is due in part to the careful selection of patients for parole and in part to the efficient supervision of patients placed on parole.

Selection of Patients for Parole

The typical method used by the New York civil State hospitals in selecting patients for parole is described by Dr. George W. Mills, superintendent of Creedmoor hospital, as follows:

"Each patient considered for parole is referred to the social service department for a preparole investigation. This covers a detailed investigation of the home environment and family group to determine the relatives' ability to provide adequate and constructive care. The attitude of members of the family toward the patient's illness, their appreciation of the situation, and their plans for his care at home are obtained. The significance of his illness and the type of supervision which he requires are explained to the relatives. The findings of the social worker's investigation are reported to the medical staff, so that the adequacy of the home care he will receive can be evaluated at the time he is presented for parole. Each patient before allowed on parole is examined by the clinical director in conference with the physician in charge of the service or at a staff meeting. Recommendations are made at this time for his treatment during his parole period. No patient is permitted to go on parole who is assaultive, destructive, homicidal, suicidal or otherwise dangerous to himself or others."

As a rule, no patient is placed on parole unless there is a safe and suitable home to receive him and a relative or friend to welcome and care for him. Positions are found, when possible, for patients who are required to earn their own living when they leave the hospital. The patient's mental condition is carefully considered by the ward physician, the clinical director and other members of the hospital staff. To be deemed eligible for parole, the patient must be harmless, tractable, and able to mingle with others without causing trouble; he must also have a fair degree of insight into his mental condition and a clear understanding of the obligations he will assume when on parole.

Supervision of Paroled Patients

The adjustment of paroled patients to community life is a cooperative undertaking in which the patient, his friends and relatives and the hospital share. The methods used by the State hospitals are the result of much thought and experience. They prove effectual in the great majority of cases. The usual procedure in such hospitals in dealing with a paroled patient is described in the following words by Dr. Russell E. Blaisdell, superintendent of Rockland State Hospital:

"The patient is paroled for a period of one year. His relatives are made aware of the supervision which is required of them in the care of the patient, and they are advised specifically concerning his care. During the parole period the patient is under the direct supervision of the social service department and he is visited at regular intervals by a social worker who interviews members of his family or other interested persons, and checks carefully on the patient's adjustment. The patient is also seen at regular intervals at a parole clinic, where he is interviewed by the parole officer and his mental reaction and physical welfare are carefully checked. At this time various suggestions are made to the patient's relatives or friends, who are also interviewed at this time. If the patient's condition indicates that his mental reaction is again becoming abnormal, the means by which he may return are specifically explained. Where the cooperation of the relatives is lacking, or when an emergency arises, the patient is returned promptly to the hospital by the hospital car. Cases requiring special supervision are seen at more frequent intervals, and in all instances where contact is made with the patient psychotherapeutic psychiatric treatment is carried out. Patients showing continued overt disorders or exhibiting any tendency to criminal conduct are returned to the hospital promptly. Special reports from time to time are requested from relatives concerning the adjustment of certain patients."

The aim of the hospital both before and after parole is to help the patient to regain his normal place as a member of the community. Treatment during the parole period is a continuation of the treatment given in the hospital and is designed to complete, so far as possible, the adjustment of the patient. In conducting the treatment, the hospital naturally considers the welfare of the community as well as that of the patient and avoids procedures that would endanger either. The large number of patients restored to normal community life and the relatively small number that commit criminal offenses indicate that the hospital methods are well planned and are producing beneficial results to the patients and communities served.

PATIENTS PAROLED FROM NEW YORK CIVIL STATE HOSPITALS AND OFFENSES COMMITTED BY THEM, YEAR ENDED JUNE 30, 1937

	Total			Binghamton			Brooklyn			Buffalo			Central Islip		
	M.	F.	T.	M.	F.	T.	M.	F.	T.	M.	F.	T.	M.	F.	T.
Patients placed on parole during fiscal year ended June 30, 1937	5,092	4,471	9,563	145	154	299	365	388	753	675	402	1,077	446	364	810
Patients returned from parole during year	2,249	1,645	3,894	49	44	93	106	115	221	581	270	851	48	55	103
Patients discharged from parole during year	2,415	2,273	4,688	78	86	164	204	239	443	138	140	278	284	210	494
Average number of patients on parole during year	2,951	2,882	5,833	105	113	218	275	317	592	142	166	308	352	276	628
Offenses committed by paroled patients during year:															
Misdemeanors	26	3	29	..	..	..	..	..	..	3	1	4	5	..	5
Felonies	11	..	11	..	..	..	..	..	..	1	..	1	..	..	..

	Creedmoor			Gowanda			Harlem Valley			Hudson River			Kings Park		
	M.	F.	T.	M.	F.	T.	M.	F.	T.	M.	F.	T.	M.	F.	T.
Patients placed on parole during fiscal year ended June 30, 1937	209	332	541	346	292	638	265	302	567	139	149	288	433	227	660
Patients returned from parole during year	83	133	216	220	185	405	100	121	221	48	44	92	158	86	244
Patients discharged from parole during year	158	219	377	90	65	155	100	198	298	97	82	179	233	102	335
Average number of patients on parole during year	146	225	371	106	83	189	137	221	358	93	113	206	295	147	442
Offenses committed by paroled patients during year:															
Misdemeanors	3	..	3	..	..	..	..	..	..	1	1	2	..	..	..
Felonies	1	..	1	..	..	..	..	..	..	..	..	..	2	..	2

PATIENTS PAROLED FROM NEW YORK CIVIL STATE HOSPITALS AND OFFENSES COMMITTED BY THEM, YEAR ENDED JUNE 30, 1937

	Manhattan			Marcy			Middletown			Pilgrim			Psy. Institute		
	M.	F.	T.	M.	F.	T.	M.	F.	T.	M.	F.	T.	M.	F.	T.
Patients placed on parole during fiscal year ended June 30, 1937	351	345	696	135	102	237	258	211	469	271	283	554	57	45	102
Patients returned from parole during year	107	114	221	47	35	82	163	106	269	88	50	138	5	10	15
Patients discharged from parole during year	233	221	454	91	76	167	73	65	138	87	84	171	70	38	108
Average number of patients on parole during year	286	257	543	100	93	193	89	98	187	131	155	286	89	33	122
Offenses committed by paroled patients during year:															
Misdemeanors	6	..	6	..	..	..	..	..	..	2	..	2	..	..	..
Felonies	..	..	..	..	..	..	..	..	..	..	..	..	..	..	..

	Rochester			Rockland			St. Lawrence			Syracuse Psy. Hospital			Utica			Willard		
	M.	F.	T.	M.	F.	T.	M.	F.	T.	M.	F.	T.	M.	F.	T.	M.	F.	T.
Patients placed on parole during fiscal year ended June 30, 1937	118	217	335	471	278	749	100	71	171	5	3	8	154	168	322	149	138	287
Patients returned from parole during year	26	33	59	225	80	305	31	8	39	5	2	7	108	104	212	51	50	101
Patients discharged from parole during year	65	96	161	206	191	397	72	47	119	..	1	1	80	64	144	56	49	105
Average number of patients on parole during year	83	136	219	246	207	453	68	59	127	..	1	1	126	117	243	81	66	147
Offenses committed by paroled patients during year:																		
Misdemeanors	..	..	..	3	1	4	..	..	..	..	..	..	3	..	3	..	..	..
Felonies	1	..	1	3	..	3	1	..	1	..	..	..	2	..	2	..	..	..

INDEX

N

O

P

SOCIAL PROBLEMS AND SOCIAL POLICY:

The American Experience

An Arno Press Collection

Bachman, George W. and Lewis Meriam. **The Issue of Compulsory Health Insurance.** 1948

Bishop, Ernest S. **The Narcotic Drug Problem.** 1920

Bosworth, Louise Marion. **The Living Wage of Women Workers.** 1911

[Brace, Emma, editor]. **The Life of Charles Loring Brace.** 1894

Brown, Esther Lucile. **Social Work as a Profession.** 4th Edition. 1942

Brown, Roy M. **Public Poor Relief in North Carolina.** 1928

Browning, Grace. **Rural Public Welfare.** 1941

Bruce, Isabel Campbell and Edith Eickhoff. **The Michigan Poor Law.** 1936

Burns, Eveline M. **Social Security and Public Policy.** 1956

Cahn, Frances and Valeska Bary. **Welfare Activities of Federal, State, and Local Governments in California, 1850-1934.** 1936

Campbell, Persia. **The Consumer Interest.** 1949

Davies, Stanley Powell. **Social Control of the Mentally Deficient.** 1930

Devine, Edward T. **The Spirit of Social Work.** 1911

Douglas, Paul H. and Aaron Director. **The Problem of Unemployment.** 1931

Eaton, Allen in Collaboration with Shelby M. Harrison. **A Bibliography of Social Surveys.** 1930

Epstein, Abraham. **The Challenge of the Aged.** 1928

Falk, I[sidore] S., Margaret C. Klem, and Nathan Sinai. **The Incidence of Illness and the Receipt and Costs of Medical Care Among Representative Families.** 1933

Fisher, Irving. **National Vitality, its Wastes and Conservation.** 1909

Freund, Ernst. **The Police Power:** Public Policy and Constitutional Rights. 1904

Gladden, Washington. **Applied Christianity:** Moral Aspects of Social Questions. 1886

Hartley, Isaac Smithson, editor. **Memorial of Robert Milham Hartley.** 1882

Hollander, Jacob H. **The Abolition of Poverty.** 1914

Kane, H[arry] H[ubbell]. **Opium-Smoking in America and China.** 1882

Klebaner, Benjamin Joseph. **Public Poor Relief in America, 1790-1860.** 1951

Knapp, Samuel L. **The Life of Thomas Eddy.** 1834

Lawrence, Charles. **History of the Philadelphia Almshouses and Hospitals from the Beginning of the Eighteenth to the Ending of the Nineteenth Centuries.** 1905

[Massachusetts Commission on the Cost of Living]. **Report of the Commission on the Cost of Living.** 1910

[Massachusetts Commission on Old Age Pensions, Annuities and Insurance]. **Report of the Commission on Old Age Pensions, Annuities and Insurance.** 1910

[New York State Commission to Investigate Provision for the Mentally Deficient]. **Report of the State Commission to Investigate Provision for the Mentally Deficient.** 1915

[Parker, Florence E., Estelle M. Stewart, and Mary Conymgton, compilers]. **Care of Aged Persons in the United States.** 1929

Pollock, Horatio M., editor. **Family Care of Mental Patients.** 1936

Pollock, Horatio M. **Mental Disease and Social Welfare.** 1941

Powell, Aaron M., editor. **The National Purity Congress;** Its Papers, Addresses, Portraits. 1896

The President's Commission on the Health Needs of the Nation. **Building America's Health.** [1952]. Five vols. in two

Prostitution in America: Three Investigations, 1902-1914. 1975

Rubinow, I[saac] M. **The Quest for Security.** 1934

Shaffer, Alice, Mary Wysor Keefer, and Sophonisba P. Breckinridge. **The Indiana Poor Law.** 1936

Shattuck, Lemuel. **Report to the Committee of the City Council Appointed to Obtain the Census of Boston for the Year 1845.** 1846

The State and Public Welfare in Nineteenth-Century America: Five Investigations, 1833-1877. 1975

Stewart, Estelle M. **The Cost of American Almshouses.** 1925

Taylor, Graham. **Pioneering on Social Frontiers.** 1930

[United States Senate Committee on Education and Labor]. **Report of the Committee of the Senate Upon the Relations Between Labor and Capital.** 1885. Four vols.

Walton, Robert P. **Marihuana, America's New Drug Problem.** 1938

Williams, Edward Huntington. **Opiate Addiction.** 1922

Williams, Pierce assisted by Isabel C. Chamberlain. **The Purchase of Medical Care Through Fixed Periodic Payment.** 1932

Willoughby, W[estal] W[oodbury]. **Opium as an International Problem.** 1925

Wisner, Elizabeth. **Public Welfare Administration in Louisiana.** 1930